Kick Butts!

A Kid's Action Guide to a Tobacco-Free America

Arlene Hirschfelder

The Scarecrow Press, Inc.
Lanham, Maryland, and London
2001

SCARECROW PRESS, INC.

Published in the United States of America
by Scarecrow Press, Inc.
4720 Boston Way, Lanham, Maryland 20706
www.scarecrowpress.com

4 Pleydell Gardens, Folkestone
Kent CT20 2DN, England

British Library Cataloguing-in-Publication Information Available

Library of Congress Cataloging-in-Publication Data

Hirschfelder, Arlene B.
    Kick butts! : a kid's action guide to a tobacco-free America / Arlene Hirschfelder.
      p. cm.
    Originally published: Parsippany, N.J. : J. Messner, 1998.
    Includes bibliographical references and index.
    ISBN 0-8108-3913-X (pbk. : alk. paper)
     1. Youth—Tobacco use—United States—Juvenile literature. 2. Cigarettes—United
States—History—Juvenile literature. 3. Tobacco habit—United States—
Prevention—Juvenile literature. 4. Tobacco habit—Treatment—United States—
Juvenile literature. [1. Tobacco habit. 2. Smoking.] I. Title.
    HV5745 .H57 2001
    613.85—dc21   00-067023

To

Dennis Hirschfelder
whose name should be on the title page next to mine

Beverly Singer
whose friendship has enriched my life

Ariane Baczynski
whose flawless research skills helped make
this book possible

Contents

Part Two: Kids Kick Butts

Tobacco products kill more than 1,100 Americans each day. Yet every day, more than 3,000 young people try their first cigarette. Of the young people who start smoking today, 23 will be murdered, 30 will die in traffic-related accidents, and 750 will die from tobacco-related

kick butts!

PART ONE

Kick Butts! A Kid's Action Guide to a Tobacco-Free America is about tobacco use in the United States. It is really two books in one. The first part describes the main events in the history of cigarettes and smokeless tobacco from the 1870s to the 1990s. You will learn interesting facts about cigarettes, such as when the first modern cigarette was "born," how the Roaring Twenties affected female smokers, and why many American soldiers returned from war hopelessly addicted to cigarettes. Here also is the history of the people who make the cigarettes and tobacco products, those who advertise them, and those who fight against tobacco.

PART TWO

The second part of *Kick Butts!* is an action guide to inspire you to stay smoke-free. Here are stories of people your age who have jumped into action and fought tobacco in a variety of ways. Young people taking action is nothing new. At the beginning of this century, young people joined anticigarette organizations, carried out "stings" to stop the illegal sale of cigarettes to minors, and wrote letters to tobacco companies. Young people are still fighting tobacco today. All over the country, they have banded together to carry out research, design smoking-education programs for young children, and create antismoking campaigns. Lots of these boys and girls have succeeded in getting laws passed. Yes, you have real power. Perhaps some of these stories will encourage you and your friends and class-mates to do something to fight tobacco, too.

diseases. These are shocking facts, but then **tobacco** is a shocking product. When used exactly as intended, **tobacco** causes addiction, disease, and early death. No other product in American history has been as controversial or as firmly rooted in our culture as **tobacco**.

Finally, kick butts!

delivers the information you need to know to become educated about tobacco. The "Tobacco Facts" and "Resources" at the back of the book give you information you can use in all kinds of presentations as well as the names and addresses of government agencies and tobacco control groups. Many of them will send you free information.

Our society won't be smoke-free until young people like you realize smoking is not cool. This book is dedicated to that goal. Now go out and "kick butts!"

Arlene Hirschfelder

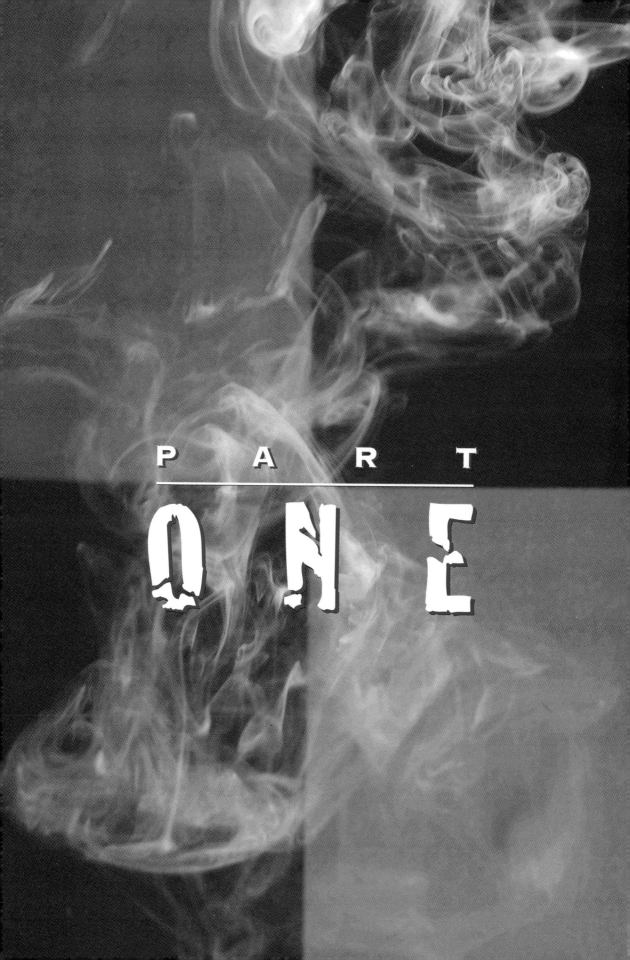

PART

ONE

The
Story
of
Tobacco
in
America

CHAPTER ONE

HAND-ROLLED TO "TAILOR-MADE"

The Cigarette Maker.

In 1870 the United States was in the middle of great change. The Civil War had ended only five years earlier, and Reconstruction would last for seven more. Many Americans were changing, too. A nation of cotton, corn, and wheat farmers was becoming a nation of factory workers and consumers. The industries that had been churning out guns and bullets for the war effort were now producing a myriad of low-priced consumer goods. The tobacco industry, like other industries, was experiencing a surge in business. Tobacco, grown mainly in Virginia and North Carolina, had been a major cash crop since colonial times. Tobacco leaves were hand-rolled into fat cigars and ground up into chew. Cigarettes were hand-rolled also, but that was about to change in the 1870s.

On January 11, 1879, a reporter for *The New York Times* wrote that "street boys who are not yet out of child's clothes snatch the discarded stubs of cigars of grown men and smoke them in imitation of their elders."

Enter the Machine

The year was 1872 when John F. Allen and Lewis Ginter, owners of a Richmond, Virginia, factory, were turning out hand-rolled cigarettes. A "roller"—usually a young woman with skillful hands—rolled four to five cigarettes a minute. That added up to about 300 cigarettes an hour. During a ten-hour workday, a roller could produce 3,000 short and slim smokes. The hand-rolled

11

cigarettes grew in popularity, and Allen and Ginter had to find a way to keep up with the demand.

They decided to sponsor a contest for the invention of a machine that could roll cigarettes automatically. The prize was a whopping $75,000!

In 1881, James Bonsack took out a patent on a design for a cigarette-rolling machine. Bonsack was a 22-year-old mechanic from Virginia whose invention poured a flow of shredded tobacco through a feeder device and then onto a thin strip of paper. The paper was rolled into a single long tube. As the tube came out of the machine, a rotary cutting knife cut it into equal lengths. Bonsack was excited at the prospect of selling his machine and allowed Allen and Ginter to try it out on a trial basis. Although the Bonsack machine could produce over 70,000 cigarettes in a ten-hour day, the two factory owners were not ready to have their factory become automated. They still believed that smokers, given a choice, would choose a hand-rolled cigarette over a machine-made one, so they rejected the machine. The Bonsack machine also had some technical problems that concerned them; the flow of shredded tobacco toward the rollers often stalled and slowed down production.

But that isn't the end of the story. In neighboring North Carolina, James Buchanan "Buck" Duke heard about the Bonsack machine. Always trusting his hunches, Duke, a 26-year-old tobacco farmer, had a strong feeling that people would buy the "tailor-mades" or manufactured cigarettes. In

1883, Duke ordered two Bonsack machines for his Durham factory but only after Bonsack and a Duke mechanic named William O'Brien had fixed the machine's technical problems. On April 30, 1884, the modern cigarette was born. That day, the Bonsack machine ran for a full ten hours and turned out 120,000 cigarettes. Duke, aware of the value of advertising, labeled his Pin Head brand with the following words: "These cigarettes are manufactured on the Bonsack Cigarette Machine."

To get people to buy his cigarettes, Duke put the smokes into colorful packs with brightly colored labels. He even inserted free gifts, such as cards of baseball players, into the packs. Baseball became the national pastime, and the players were the celebrities of the day. Soon, collecting cigarette cards became a craze for young and old. Duke also placed ads in newspapers and magazines, on

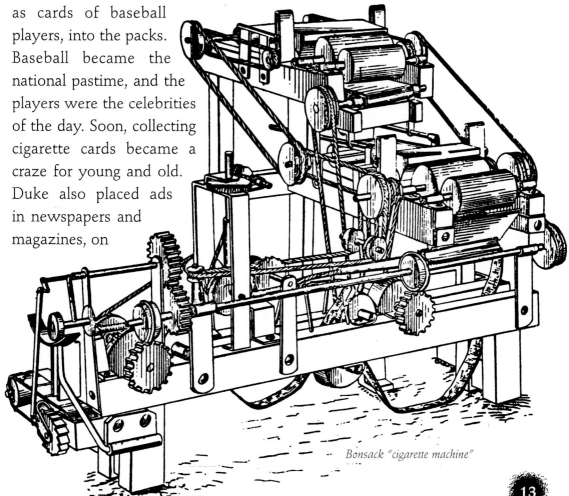

Bonsack "cigarette machine"

13

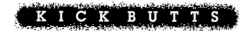

KICK BUTTS

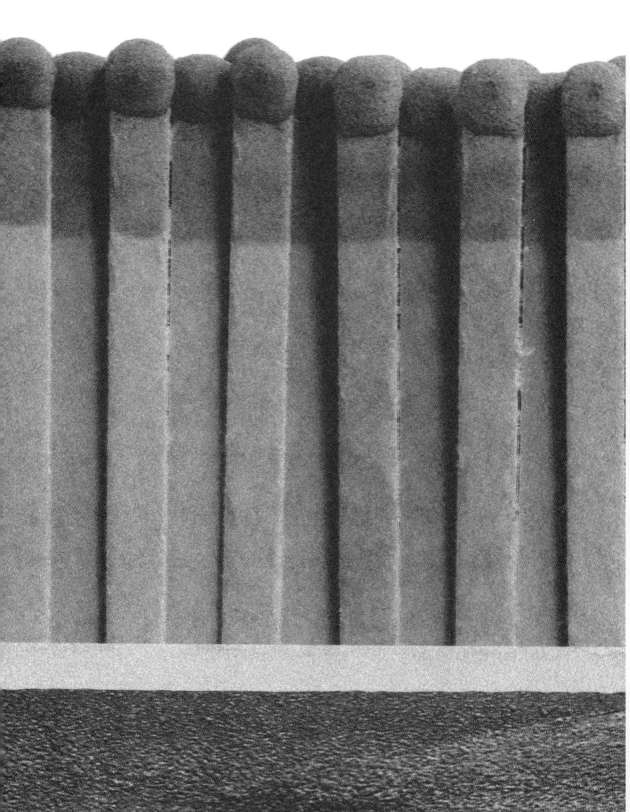

billboards, in theater programs, and on posters tacked to fences, walls, and storefronts. In 1889, Duke spent $800,000 on advertising for the 834 million cigarettes his factory manufactured that year! He set a trend that would shake up the tobacco industry. Duke cigarette sales went up and up, and competing companies soon copied his methods.

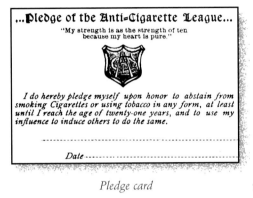

Pledge card

...**Pledge of the Anti-Cigarette League**...

"My strength is as the strength of ten because my heart is pure."

I do hereby pledge myself upon honor to abstain from smoking Cigarettes or using tobacco in any form, at least until I reach the age of twenty-one years, and to use my influence to induce others to do the same.

Date ----

Another invention helped boost the popularity of cigarettes. In 1892, Joshua Pusey, a lawyer from Lima, Pennsylvania, made the first portable cardboard matchbook. It held fifty matches. Before the arrival of the cardboard matchbook—which was also disposable—smokers had to carry wooden matches lin metal waterproof containers. At first, Pusey's invention failed because he put the striking surface on the inside of the matchbook. Sparks created by the friction from one match often ignited the others, scorching the users' fingertips. Discouraged, Pusey sold his invention to the Diamond Match Company in 1895. The company fixed the problem by placing the striking surface on the outside. Once the matchbook was safer to use, Diamond was able to sell it in the hundreds of thousands. Now smokers—could easily and cheaply light up whenever and wherever they wished. And they did.

In 1893, Charles B. Hubbell, president of the New York City Board of Education, began a crusade against cigarettes in public schools. He decided to form an anticigarette-smoking league in every boys' school in the city. When a boy joined, he signed a pledge not to smoke until he was 21. He received a diamond-shaped badge of solid silver whose face bore the words "The cigarette must go." The boys took great pride in living up to their pledges. If a member was caught smoking, he turned in his badge and was barred from the league for six months. After he returned, he got his badge back and was given another chance to be a member. Eventually 25,000 New York schoolboys belonged to the leagues established in almost all of the 63 male grammar schools in the city.

Getting Angry About Smoking

Not everyone was pleased about the widespread popularity and availability of cigarettes, however. Parents were the most upset by youthful puffing. They warned their children that smoking would lead to stunted growth and medical problems such as weak lungs. Principals and teachers were equally upset by children who smoked. They saw how boys and girls who smoked neglected their studies and skipped school. But what bothered educators the most was cigarette advertising. It made young people want to buy smokes. Ads came in the form of gimmicks such as cards, buttons, flags, and other free gifts tucked into cigarette packs. The young people wanted the giveaways, and many would do anything to get them. Some kids stole money from their parents to get the tobacco and the freebies.

State lawmakers became worried about the effect of cigarette advertising on the young, and their anger led to a series of laws. In the 1890s, twenty-six states passed laws prohibiting the sale or giving away of cigarettes to minors. But there was a hitch. The term *minor*, referring to someone under-age, meant different things in different states. In some states, it referred to those under 16; in others, it referred to those under 21. Well over half the state legislatures (there were 44 states in the Union at the time) tried to keep young nonsmokers from smoking. In New York, for example, lawmakers made it a misdemeanor for youngsters under 16 to smoke in public. But state laws forbidding the sale of cigarettes to minors were fairly useless, and enforcing the antismoking laws was nearly impossible. Cigarette sellers kept right on attracting young customers. Eight- and nine-year-old children went into stores and bought cigarettes, without any questions from the shopkeepers. Some shopkeepers even broke open packs of cigarettes and sold single cigarettes, called "loosies," to the young smokers. The same thing still goes on today.

Not all young people were interested in smoking. Many followed the lead of people like Lucy Page Gaston, one of the many private citizens who were busy organizing antitobacco crusades. In 1899 she won the support of businesses in Chicago and founded the Chicago Anti-Cigarette League. The League set up clinics to help smokers quit the habit. Children were encouraged to take a pledge not to smoke. In addition, youngsters who took the pledge were asked to patrol the streets of their neighborhoods. If they saw adults smoking, the youngsters snatched the cigarettes from their lips. Special officers were hired by the League to arrest anyone under 18 who was found smoking in public.

The war for a smoke-free AMERICA was on.

CHAPTER TWO

TOBACCO COMPANIES GET BIGGER

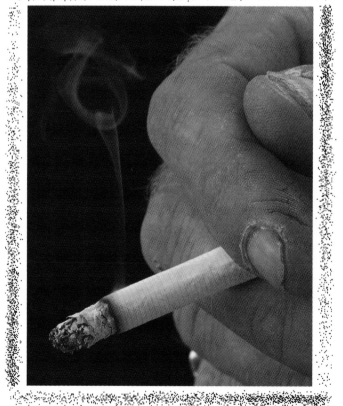

The United States at the beginning of the twentieth century was truly a nation on the go. President Theodore Roosevelt, physically fit and a nonsmoker, epitomized the active and youthful spirit of the times. America's power was growing overseas, and the economy was booming at home. Between 1897 and 1904, over 4,000 companies combined to form 257 large corporations. These enormous combinations of companies, called trusts, worked together to crush competition and control prices in the steel, oil, railroad, sugar, meatpacking, and tobacco industries. Big business had arrived in a big way.

The American Tobacco Company was founded by James Duke around 1890. During the 1880s and 1890s, he spent huge sums of money to make his company bigger and richer. Duke bought up at least two hundred fifty smaller tobacco companies and paid his competitors to get out of the tobacco business. By 1904 the American Tobacco Company was almost a monopoly. That is, it was a gigantic company that made 88 percent of the nation's cigarettes, 80 percent of its chewing tobacco, 75 percent of its pipe tobacco, and over 90 percent of its snuff—powdered or finely cut tobacco either loose or wrapped in a pouch. Such a stranglehold on one industry angered President Roosevelt. In 1907 the President directed the Attorney General to file suit against the American Tobacco Company and 64 other defendants for violating the Antitrust Act of 1890. This law outlawed monopolies. It wasn't the huge profits of the tobacco companies that

In 1902 and 1903, children wrote letters to the American Tobacco Company, begging the company to stop making cigarettes.

*"**Gentlemen:** I am a boy of Chicago, and today's paper says that the Hotel Somerset burned and four lives were lost all on account of one cigarette thrown carelessly on a boy fiend's bed. Don't you think the boys' lives are worth more than your profits? I beg you to stop the manufacturing of cigarettes."*—Earl Cunningham, Chicago, Illinois

*"**Gentlemen:** Have you ever thought how many boys and girls you have killed by cigars and cigarettes? You would be better off morally if you would take my advice and quit it and go into some business that is more honorable."*—Jennie Wilson, Clyde, Ohio

In the late 1800s, Allen & Ginter of Richmond, Virginia, put small picture cards in each cigarette box to get people to buy their product. Their sales zoomed, and other companies picked up the gimmick. Subjects pictured included birds, flags, and baseball players. One card set issued in 1909 included a card of Honus Wagner, a Pittsburgh Pirates' shortstop. This card is now the most desirable in the sports card world. As the story goes, Wagner opposed cigarette smoking and did *not* want his photo used to endorse cigarettes, especially to children. He insisted the cards be taken out of circulation, but several dozen remained. These cards are now extremely valuable. In 1996 a New York auction house sold a Honus Wagner card in mint condition for $640,000!

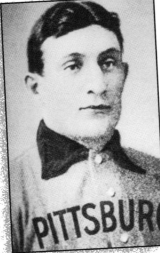

Honus Wagner

bothered Roosevelt. Rather, it was their greed and irresponsibility that angered him. "We draw the line against misconduct, not against wealth," Theodore Roosevelt declared.

The trial began in 1908 and took three years to conclude. In 1911 the Supreme Court ordered Duke to break up his company into smaller firms. The companies that American Tobacco had swallowed up were set free to compete against it. Roosevelt's antitrust policy did not end the power of the giant tobacco companies, but it did increase the role of governmental regulation. During Roosevelt's presidency, Congress passed the Pure Food and Drug Act of 1906. This law protected Americans from dangerous drugs and chemicals that might be put in their medicines, foods, and drinks. Today, the Food and Drug Administration (FDA) that found its beginnings in the 1906 act wants the authority to regulate nicotine in tobacco as a drug. The regulation of businesses continued during the presidency of Woodrow Wilson. In 1914, Congress passed the Federal Trade Commission Act. This act set up the Federal Trade Commission (FTC) and gave it the authority to investigate and publish reports about business activities. Today, the FTC polices businesses and protects consumers from deceptive business practices, such as a dishonest claim or promise in an advertisement.

SILK GIVEAWAY

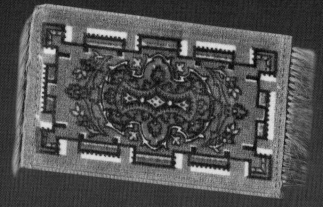

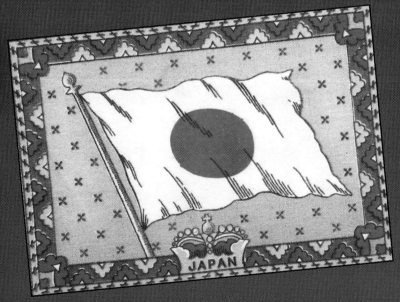

Around 1912, tobacco companies inserted small silk rectangles in cigarette boxes in the hope of attracting female smokers. Women bought the cigarettes and collected the "silks," which they stitched together and sewed onto pillows and bedspreads. Small silk, rugs were also the perfect size for a child's dollhouse.

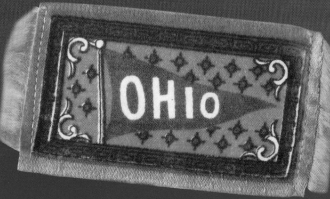

A Famous Brand Is Born

Despite the breakup of the American Tobacco Company into smaller, competing companies, nothing really changed in the way the tobacco industry did business. Four major tobacco companies continued to manufacture, advertise, and sell their products to American consumers. In 1913 a new brand of cigarettes was born when the R. J. Reynolds Tobacco Company introduced Camels. This brand was the first to feature the "modern" blended cigarette. It contained Turkish and home-grown tobaccos. The company chose the name "Camel" to suggest the Middle Eastern origin of the tobacco leaf. The brand's logo is one of the most famous of any product in the United States. The story of how the camel got on the package is an interesting one.

Just as the R. J. Reynolds package designers were looking around for a model of a camel to copy for Camels, the Barnum and Bailey Circus came to Winston-Salem, North Carolina, the home of R. J. Reynolds. One of the stars of the circus was "Old Joe," a one-humped camel from Arabia. Always searching for new ideas to advertise its products, the tobacco company sent an employee to take a picture of the camel. The package designer used the photograph of Old Joe to make a drawing for the cigarette pack, and an artist added the pyramids and palm trees for special effect.

Advertising history was made—that same image still appears on Camel cigarettes today. On October 21, 1913, R. J. Reynolds launched the first national cigarette advertising campaign. It cost millions of dollars and made Camels the number-one-selling cigarette in just six short years.

Not to be outdone, the American Tobacco Company introduced Lucky Strike cigarettes in 1916. The name actually dates from 1856: "Lucky Strike" was the name of a chewing tobacco used by gold miners in California and silver miners in Colorado. The ad campaign for Lucky Strike cigarettes showed a piece of toast with a fork through it accompanied by the slogan "Lucky Strike, It's Toasted."

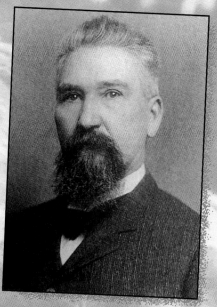

R. J. Reynolds

Tobacco Goes to War

Camels and Lucky Strike, appeared at a significant time in America's history. War broke out in Europe in 1914 and involved almost all of the major powers. At first, the United States tried to stay out of the conflict. But in April 1917, Congress declared war on Germany. By 1918, patriotic posters of American "doughboys" in the trenches appeared across the country. The art often showed a young soldier with a cigarette clenched between his teeth.

Many young men went into World War I as nonsmokers, but they didn't stay that way for long. They received free packs of cigarettes from

23

On August 6, 1913, in New York City, a squad of boys ranging in age from ten to twelve conducted a "sting" of neighborhood stores. They were able to buy cigarettes from 200 shopkeepers. The law required that no cigarettes be sold to children under sixteen, so the boys turned the names of the lawbreakers over to the East Side Protective Association. Today, over 80 years later, kids still conduct stings all over the nation, proving that stores still sell cigarettes to minors (a person under 18 years of age).

the Red Cross, the Salvation Army, and the YMCA. The army also encouraged the use of tobacco by giving cigarettes to the soldiers with their daily food rations. When deciding which cigarettes to provide to the troops, the government awarded contracts to the cigarette manufacturers based on their sales at home before the war. Because Camels were the best-selling cigarette at the time, most soldiers received that brand.

Why were cigarettes popular at the front? A Massachusetts reporter wrote that soldiers in the trenches needed cigarettes to "soothe the nerves . . . and help [them] endure the strain [of combat]." But others knew the addictive quality of tobacco. Hudson Maxim, an explosives expert and inventor, predicted the effect of smoking when he said, "cigarette smoking will be responsible for a larger number of deaths than the poisonous gases of the Germans . . . because while the German gases affect the body, they do not, like the cigarette, impair [hurt] the mind." When the fighting stopped, in November 1918, the soldiers began to return home. Some smoked and some did not. Many who continued to smoke had already become addicted to cigarettes.

1910 Antismoking poster ▶

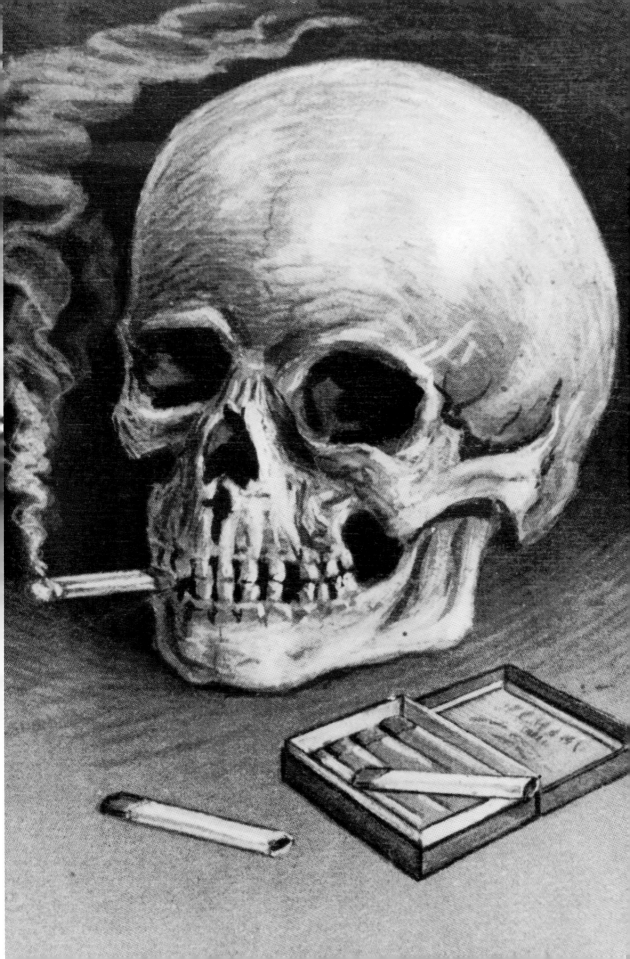

CHAPTER THREE

TOBACCO TARGETS WOMEN

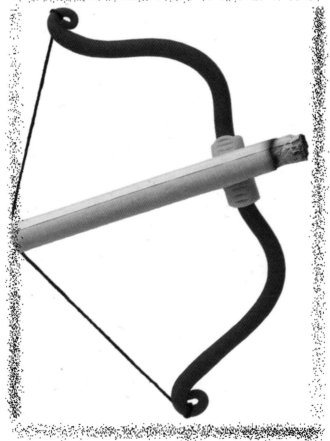

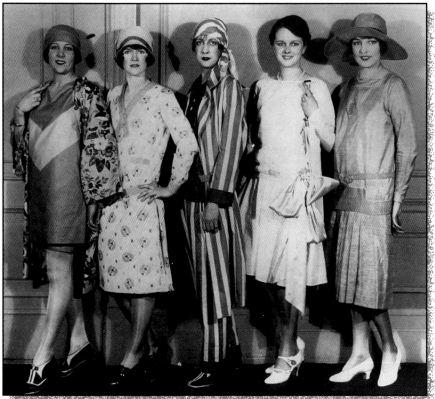

Women in the early 1900s

If a woman smoked cigarettes during the late 1800s and early 1900s, she could expect trouble with a capital *T*. It wasn't acceptable behavior for women at the turn of the century. A woman who smoked was regarded as morally "loose," unfeminine, and maybe even insane. Some women did smoke in private, but smoking in public was unheard of. In fact, some cities, such as New York, made it illegal for women to smoke in public. Young female smokers could be expelled from school if caught puffing on a cigarette.

Many women were opposed to smoking. As

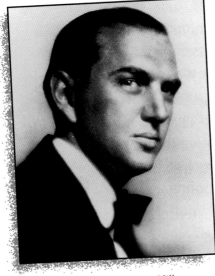

George Washington Hill

On July 7, 1923, the California Department of Agriculture sent out a statement that some cattle got into a tobacco field, ate the plants, and died before morning. Within a few days, 21 more died from "chewing the weed." The department's statement added, ". . .The wonder is that 25 or 30 million smokers in the United States are so blind that they cannot see that a drug that will kill cows is not the sort of thing to make men manly and efficient."

City debutantes who strolled down that city's Fifth Avenue on Easter Sunday, holding and smoking cigarettes. The parade made front-page news all over the nation. And soon women in other cities began to smoke on the street, too.

The tobacco companies added other gimmicks to cigarettes to make them appealing to women. Marlboros were made with a red "fashion" tip designed to blend in with the smoker's lipstick. One of the most successful and profitable ads in the history of the tobacco industry appeared in 1928 for the American Tobacco Company. Albert Lasker, advertising executive, launched the Lucky Strike ad campaign with the slogan "Reach for a Lucky Instead of a Sweet." The ad suggested to women that cigarette smoking would help them slim down and stay thin. The story goes that the idea for the ad was based on a hunch Lasker had when he saw two women, one slim and smoking a cigarette, and the other stout and eating a piece of candy. The candy companies were furious with the Lucky Strike ad and asserted that cigarettes and not candy were actually harmful to one's health. The FTC stepped in and told the tobacco companies not to advertise cigarettes as weight-reducing devices. But it was too late! Women had already bought the powerful message. In their minds, it was easier to stay thin by smoking than by exercising. The Lucky

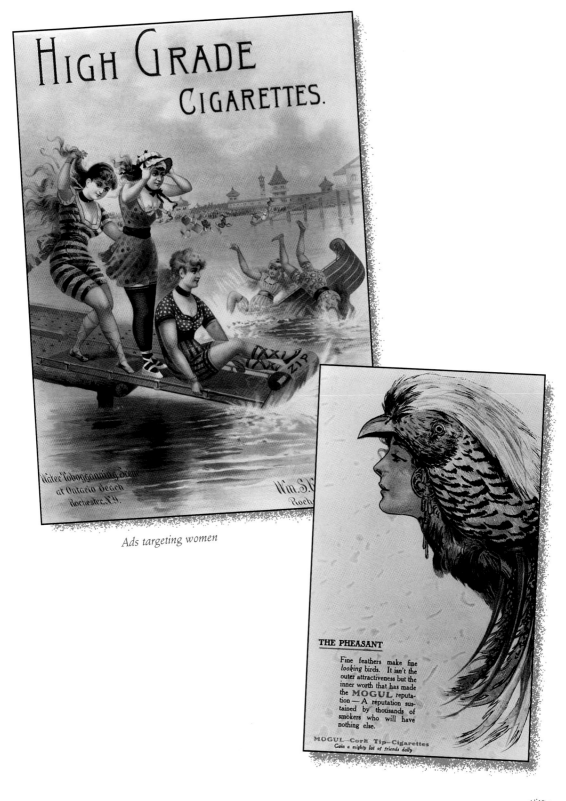

Ads targeting women

THE PHEASANT

Fine feathers make fine *looking* birds. It isn't the outer attractiveness but the inner worth that has made the MOGUL reputation — A reputation sustained by thousands of smokers who will have nothing else.

MOGUL—Cork Tip—Cigarettes
Gain a mighty lot of friends daily

Strike ad campaign helped increase the American Tobacco Company's profits from $21 million in 1925 to $46 million in 1931!

A Powerful New Medium

The 1920s also ushered in the idea of "leisure time." Labor-saving machines were relieving Americans of much of the hard physical work at home and on the job. As a result, families had more time and money to spend taking vacations, going to the movies, and using the latest technology. That technology included telephones, Kodak cameras, and the radio. The radio proved to be a powerful new medium for transmitting advertising, and the tobacco companies were right there to use it.

In August 1922, New York radio station WEAF offered ten minutes of radio time to anyone willing to pay $100. A Long Island real estate company responded to the offer and bought time for the first commercial in broadcasting history. Other companies were quick to recognize the value of radio advertising. The American Tobacco Company saw the importance of the new medium in capturing new smokers and was one of the first tobacco companies to advertise on radio. G. W. Hill created the Lucky Strike Dance Orchestra in 1928. While people enjoyed the music, they were fed ads for cigarettes. Two months after Lucky Strike commercials were first heard on radio, sales had grown by 47 percent! Other cigarette companies soon joined the move to radio. The Sir Walter

On March 5, 1924, the Michigan Supreme Court upheld the expulsion of Alice Tanton, a smoker and student at Michigan State Normal College. Tanton had started smoking before she entered college and continued to smoke while there. She also smoked in town and in public. After she was tossed out of school, Tanton sued the college president on the grounds that her personal freedom had been violated. She lost the case.

Raleigh Revue, another music show, squeezed 70 references to Raleighs, the sponsoring cigarette, into one hour of airtime.

Not everyone was happy about the growing presence of cigarette advertising. *Good Housekeeping* magazine wrote in 1929 about the danger that radio cigarette ads posed for women listeners: " . . . the use of the radio for . . . cigarette propaganda should be stopped. Parents who do not want their daughters to become cigarette fiends should be able to have a radio in their homes without feeling that they are opening their homes to a flood of . . . cigarette propaganda." Radio listeners had to wait until 1971 before cigarette advertising finally disappeared from the airwaves.

The Roaring Twenties ended with a crash. On October 29, 1929, prices on the New York Stock Exchange fell disastrously in very heavy trading. Stocks that had sold for $20 and $30 a share a few weeks before were dumped for pennies as panicky investors rushed to sell. The great depression had begun.

In November of 1924, *Reader's Digest* ran an article entitled "Does Tobacco Injure the Human Body?" in which Dr. J. Kellogg called tobacco a "heart poison." *Reader's Digest* has been running articles about the dangers of smoking ever since. In fact, *Reader's Digest* should win a prize for the number of times it has published articles about the hazards of smoking. Over 100 articles on the issue of smoking and health have appeared in the magazine.

CHAPTER FOUR

TOUGH TIMES

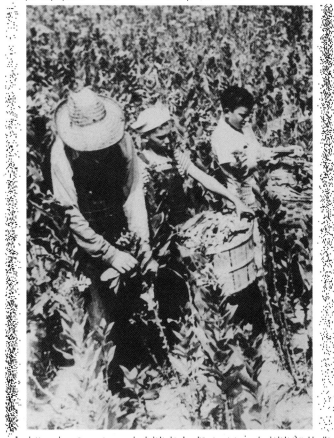

Tough times for tobacco farmers

Over five thousand banks lost money in the 1929 stock market crash and had to close their doors. Peoples' savings had disappeared almost overnight. Unable to pay their bills, huge numbers of stores and factories went bankrupt. Those businesses that managed to keep their doors open let some employees go and cut back the wages of those who remained.

Tobacco Farmers Struggle

Farmers were hard hit, too. The tough times of the 1930s were just a continuation of the nightmare that had begun in the 1920s. Growing and harvesting corn and tobacco cost more than farmers received for selling the crops. In fact, farmers were growing more food than people could afford to buy. Crop prices were dropping, but expenses were rising. The farmers tried to drive prices up by resorting to sabotage. They dumped milk into ditches, burned corn, allowed wheat to rot in the fields, and cut back tobacco production.

Hard times and the inaction of President Herbert Hoover had a big impact on the 1932 election. Voters brought in Franklin Delano Roosevelt as president. In the famous "One Hundred Days" after Roosevelt's inauguration, Congress passed the New Deal legislation Roosevelt wanted.

In 1933, Philip Morris cigarettes were introduced. To help advertise its product, the company hired Johnny Roventini, a 22-year-old, 43-inch-tall bellhop from Brooklyn. He became the radio voice for Philip Morris cigarettes. "Call for Phil-lip Mor-ris" rang out on top radio programs, at conventions, and at ballgames during the 1930s and 1940s.

In "Why I Do Not Smoke," an essay published in the *Union Signal* on April 14, 1934, William H. Phelps explained his decision: "As it is now, I can talk intelligently with a man for five minutes without nervously reaching for a cigarette. . . . Always afraid of fire, I dread the fearful toll of cigarette stubs. . . . I would be afraid that the boys and girls of the neighborhood would imitate my habits and for their sake I do not smoke. "

The New Deal was a group of government programs designed to help America recover from the Great Depression.

Some New Deal programs were aimed at rescuing farmers. On May 12, 1933, Roosevelt signed the Agricultural Adjustment Act (AAA) to provide immediate relief to growers of "basic" crops such as wheat, corn, cotton, and tobacco. For example, tobacco farmers were offered government payments if they volunteered *not* to grow tobacco. By cutting back their production, tobacco farmers hoped to drive up prices. In February 1936, the Soil Conservation and Domestic Allotment Act replaced the AAA. Under this act, farmers were urged to stop growing crops that used up too many nutrients from the soil. Such crops included cotton, tobacco, corn, and wheat. Two years later, however, the agreement by farmers to restrict tobacco production broke down, and farmers planted thousands more acres of tobacco. The crop flooded the market, and prices fell. To stabilize crop prices and farmers' incomes, Congress passed the Agricultural Adjustment Act of 1938. The law set quotas on the number of acres of tobacco that farmers could plant.

Radio Days

Somehow, people found ways to survive the Depression. Radio programs helped them overcome feelings of helplessness and despair. Families gathered around their radios to laugh at the antics of comedian Jack Benny or be scared by mysteries

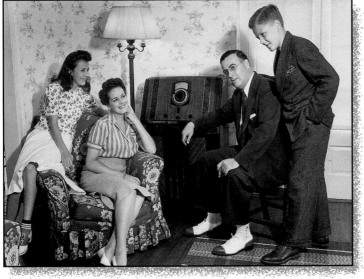

Family listening to 1940s radio broadcast

such as *The Shadow.* Along with the popular dance tunes, jokes, and whodunits came a steady flow of advertisements. Tobacco companies continued to pour millions of dollars into radio commercials. American Tobacco's Lucky Strike brand sponsored one of the most popular music programs of the time. The *Lucky Strike Hit Parade* started on radio in 1928 and continued into the 1950s, when it crossed over into television. In 1938, the show reached a new peak in its popularity when producers introduced a sweepstakes promotion in which free cartons of Luckies were given away to anyone who guessed each week's three most popular tunes. Nearly 7 million entries were sent in each week. Each of the major tobacco companies had a music show, featuring either a big band such as Tommy Dorsey's (hired by Brown & Williamson) or the singing Andrew Sisters (hired by Liggett & Myers). Liggett & Myers, the makers of Chesterfields, tried to put popular singer Bing Crosby on the payroll, but he didn't last long. Crosby was fired because he refused to say on the air, "Don't forget to buy your mother a carton of Chesterfields on Mother's Day." Crosby's mother hated smoking.

Cigarette advertisements continued to appear on billboards, in magazines, and in daily newspapers during the Depression. By 1930, the American Tobacco Company, Brown & Williamson, and other tobacco companies were spending piles of money on print advertising. Often, the ads featured famous people doing exciting things and praising the cigarettes. An endless stream of baseball players, golfers, tennis stars, and even Olympic champions mouthed such Camel slogans as "They Don't Get Your Wind" or "Never Get on Your Nerves." Women, especially celebrities and movie stars, were featured in many tobacco print ads of the 1930s. Amelia Earhart, the famous pilot, promoted Lucky Strikes. So did Carole Lombard, a popular actress. Camels pictured all kinds of women in their ads: college students, housewives, office workers, and factory workers.

To lure more and more people into buying cigarettes, tobacco companies suggested that doctors, the final authorities on health issues, approved of smoking. Camels showed a doctor holding a pack. Philip Morris ads said tests by groups of doctors "proved conclusively that in changing to

The following news item appeared in South Dakota's *Waukonda Monitor* in early 1935: "Picked by the nation's 4-H clubs as the healthiest boy in America, Leland Monasmith, eighteen, of Jerauld County, has spurned an offer to permit the use of his name in the cigarette advertising of a nationally known tobacco company, even though he admits he needs financial aid to start his college career."

Philip Morris, every case of irritation due to smoking cleared completely or definitely improved." Chesterfield ads stated that a "medical specialist" examined a group of people who smoked only Chesterfields for six months. This "specialist" concluded that their ears, noses, throats, and other organs "were not adversely affected."

Not all doctors rushed to endorse cigarettes, however. In 1933, one New Jersey medical journal criticized doctors for their careless behavior: "Hundreds of medical men have stooped to contribute their testimonials as to the harmlessness or desirability of certain brands of cigarettes, without even stopping for a moment to consider the toxic effect of any tobacco upon our American [teenagers].

In 1938, Congress gave the Federal Trade Commission the authority to regulate "unfair or deceptive acts or practices in commerce." The FTC targeted deceptive cigarette advertising and, over a 30-year period, forced cigarette makers to withdraw misleading claims 25 times.

CHAPTER FIVE

AMERICANS GO TO WAR, AND TOBACCO IS THERE

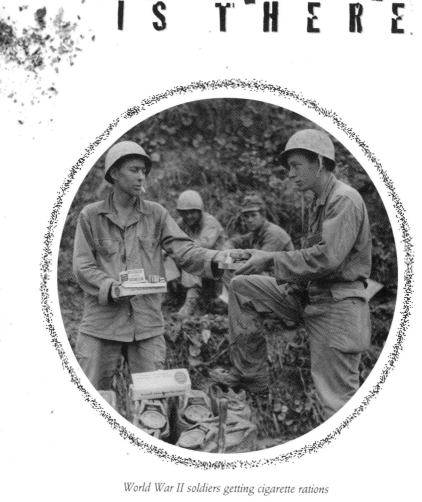

World War II soldiers getting cigarette rations

Americans were still in the midst of the Great Depression when World War II broke out in Europe in 1939. At first, President Franklin Roosevelt tried to keep the nation neutral. Our noninvolvement did not last long, however. On December 7, 1941, Japanese bombers attacked Pearl Harbor, the major United States naval base in Hawaii. The next day, President Roosevelt asked a special joint session of Congress to declare war against Japan. Congress did and soon Japan's allies, Germany and Italy, issued declarations of war on the United States. Just over a week after Pearl Harbor, the President signed the draft law that sent thousands of men to war in Europe, the Mediterranean, and the Pacific regions.

About the same time as the war started, a survey showed that 48 percent of American men and 36 percent of American women were smoking. Those figures rose sharply during World War II. Several tobacco manufacturers stepped up production so that they could increase shipments of cigarettes to military forces in combat zones. One company even added night shifts so that it could fill more orders. Cigarette production increased by almost 50 percent from 1941 to 1945—the years of America's involvement in World War II. During those years, about 20 percent of the cigarettes made in the United States were shipped to soldiers overseas, creating a shortage at home.

As in World War I, thousands of young men went to war as nonsmokers but came home addicted. Tobacco companies encouraged GIs

In a letter to *Scholastic* magazine, dated January 27, 1941, D. S. Lauver, principal of Partridge High School in Kansas, told how he had fought against tobacco for 30 years. He blamed World War I for worsening the cigarette habit: "When we sent our boys to the World War, we let the tobacco trust put cigarettes in their mouths and helped in the process by giving it our approval for its usefulness in 'quieting the nerves' in the strenuous life of the army. Ever since that time the habit has grown worse . . . ."

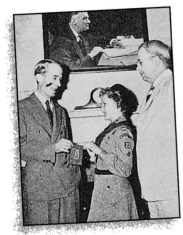

Secretary to President Roosevelt receives bag

In July 1942, Girl Scouts in Oregon came up with a plan to help check forest fires. They made 50,000 small red cloth bags, closed by a drawstring. The bags were large enough to hold a package of cigarettes and a few matches. Each time a smoker entered forest lands, a Girl Scout handed the person a bag. The theory behind the bags was that when a person reached for a cigarette, he or she would have to open the bag to get it. The action would remind the smoker to be careful with matches and cigarettes. A label on the bag explained the theory.

(members of the armed forces during World War II) to take up the smoking habit. To make sure they did, the companies provided a constant flow of free cigarettes to the troops. "Smokes" were given with K rations, balanced meals for troops in the field. Cigarettes were also provided by church groups, labor unions, and the Red Cross.

The free cigarettes contributed to the massive growth of smoking. Advertising also did its bit. Americans were spending more hours listening to the radio during the war than in any other time. The tobacco advertisers knew this and added their messages directly into radio programs. Lucky Strike ads had been on the airwaves for years, but in the fall of 1942, they took on a new character. Millions of Americans heard a radio broadcaster announce "Lucky Strike Green (pause for a trumpet blast and drum roll) Has Gone to War!" In six weeks, sales grew 38 percent.

Hello, Television

Television was just an interesting experiment in the 1930s, but by 1942, there were ten commercial stations on the "talking screens."

Permitted by the FTC to advertise on television as of 1941, the tobacco companies took full advantage of television's power as a visual communicator. In 1947, Lucky Strike began sponsoring college football games. To be a sponsor meant paying for the airtime needed to broadcast the event to viewers. Other cigarette companies did the same

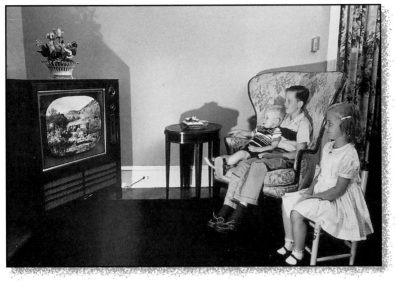

Watching TV in the 1950s

thing. Beginning in 1948, Camel sponsored the *Camel News Caravan,* the first regular news program to be sponsored across the country.

People in White Coats

Cigarette advertisers knew that people trusted doctors to tell them what was good or bad for them. So real doctors—or people dressed up in white coats to look like doctors—were paid to appear in ads to say smoking was good for the public. If one believed the ads, then one believed that Camels helped digestion, Pall Malls protected throats from irritation, and Kools protected against colds. During the 1940s and 1950s, advertisers said "science" and "research" proved the medical superiority of one brand over others. Finally, the American Medical Association (AMA) took a firm

Factory workers during World War II

stand on smoking and advertising. This national physicians' organization disliked linking doctors with smoking. In 1954 the AMA banned cigarette ads from its prestigious journal and eleven of its publications. But many Americans were misled into believing that cigarette smoking was not only not harmful but could actually be good for them.

Health was not the only message tobacco companies used to sell cigarettes. They created advertising campaigns that linked smoking with courage in battle and patriotism in general. Camel ads showed men in submarines, breaking through barbed-wire barriers, lugging antitank guns. Pall Mall used military themes in its advertising. Raleighs offered cheap prices on gift cigarettes sent to soldiers overseas.

Her Cigarette

Tobacco companies paid attention to women as well during the war years. The U.S. government suggested it was the patriotic duty of women to help the war effort. About 350,000 women responded and joined the Women's Army Corps (WAC) and the women's branch of the Navy (WAVES, or Women Accepted for Voluntary Emergency Service). At home, thousands of women joined factory assembly lines in heavy industry and defense plants to replace the men who were fighting overseas.

To the cigarette makers, women in industry were important potential customers. During the early 1940s, cigarette companies appealed to women by advertising in all the major women's magazines. Ads showing women hard at work in the war effort were designed to suggest they could smoke, do a man's job, and still be feminine. In their "Workers in the War Effort" campaign, Chesterfields displayed a smiling woman worker, cigarette hanging from her lips, dressed in blue dungarees, her helmet tilted backward. Half sticking out of her dungarees pocket is an open pack of Chesterfields, and across her body is a banner proclaiming "For My Taste It's Chesterfield."

Many young men and women who began smoking in the service or during their war work kept up the habit in civilian life. After the war, women gave up their war-related jobs and returned home to take up their lives as homemakers and mothers. There was one important change, however. The wife and mother was now probably a smoker. Many men who took up smoking during their period of service got hooked on nicotine and continued to smoke when the fighting stopped. After years of smoking, some of these smokers began to complain of persistent coughing, difficulty in breathing, chronic bronchitis, and more. In 1958, the U.S. Public Health Service released the results of a study of about 200,000 World War I and World War II veterans between the ages of 50 and 70. It showed that smokers who averaged two or more packs a day had death rates that were twice that of nonsmokers!

In 1949, candy stores in South Dakota sold candy cigarettes in packages that strongly resembled Camel, Chesterfield, and Lucky Strike packages. At the time, it was illegal for youngsters under twenty-one to buy or smoke cigarettes. A newspaper writer commented that "this candy manufacturer who is making these imitation cigarettes, the store keepers who sell them, and the people backing the South Dakota campaign to make sales of cigarettes to 16-year-old-boys and girls legal are all deserving of the unbounded contempt of every decent citizen. These envoys of evil are doing their best to make nicotine addicts—dope fiends—of every boy and girl in this country."

CHAPTER SIX

THE FILTERED FIFTIES

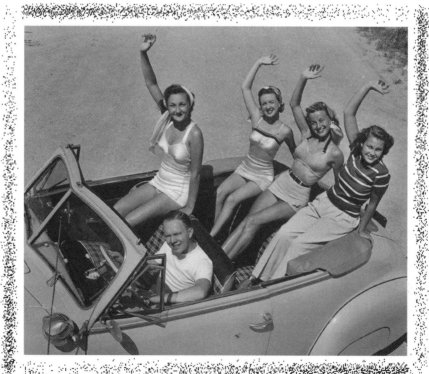

College kids of the fifties

The United States came out of World War II a powerful nation. Unlike the other nations who fought in the war, the United States had not seen its cities, countryside, and people bombed. Most Americans had a sense that all was well in the United States under the leadership of President Dwight D. Eisenhower, a wartime general and hero. The U.S. economy was in good shape, too. After enduring years of economic hardship and war, Americans in the 1950s were eager to spend money. And spend they did—on cars, new houses, and television sets.

Television became a major influence in American life during this period. By the late 1950s, 75 percent of all American families owned at least one television set.

The tobacco companies poured money into television advertising because they were certain that television sold their products better than radio, magazines, and other media. Spending went from $40 million in 1957 to about $115 million in 1961. The tobacco companies were right. Cigarette sales and profits increased.

"If you smoke a pack a day you inhale 400 milligrams of nicotine a week, which, in a single injection, would kill you quick as a bullet."—

Dr. Raymond Pearl, Reader's Digest, *January 1950*

Bad-News Mice

Despite its love of the new medium as an advertising tool, the tobacco industry faced some problems. One of these was the need to rework the health messages it had been using to sell cigarettes in the 1930s and 1940s. News from numerous scientific studies informed the public that cigarette smoking was linked to lung cancer and other serious

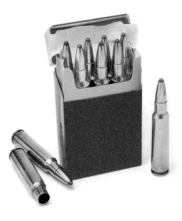

A 1958 study at North High School in Des Moines, Iowa, showed that students who did not smoke got better grades than those who smoked. The grade point average of 81 nonsmokers was considerably higher than the average of the 23 who smoked.

diseases. During 1953 and 1954, researchers at New York's Memorial Center for Cancer and Allied Diseases announced that they had produced cancer in mice by injecting them with tar condensed from cigarette smoke.

Other health reports appeared at around the same time. *Consumer Reports* published a report on the tar and nicotine content of cigarette smoke and other health hazards of smoking. Dr. Alton Ochsner, a famous surgeon, reported an increase of lung cancer due to a cancer-producing factor in cigarette smoking. The news rattled people. They got scared and stopped buying cigarettes. Faced with declining profits, the cigarette makers began to push filter-tipped cigarettes. Filter tips were nothing new. They had been around since the 1800s, when cork mouthpieces served as filters. In the late 1930s, Viceroys introduced hollow cardboard tubes filled with cotton tufts and folded wads of paper. In the 1950s, tobacco companies revived filters to reassure smokers it was okay to keep on smoking.

In 1952, the first filter-tipped cigarette to be promoted in a big way was Kent, named after Herbert A. Kent, a J. P. Lorillard executive. A massive print and television advertising campaign hailed Kents as the "Greatest Health Protection in Cigarette History." It was a clear response to the health scare. Kent ads boasted a new "micronite" filter tip that took out "more nicotine and tars than any other leading cigarette." Smokers found Kents hard to smoke, so the filters were loosened up. This made them easier to smoke, but nicotine and tar levels went up. In 1957, without publicity, Kent abandoned its original micronite filter.

After Kent filter tips appeared on the market, other cigarette makers went to work to develop competing filters. Filter brands multiplied, and the competing brands all claimed the best combination of good taste with low tar and nicotine. In 1957, filter tips accounted for almost 50 percent of all cigarette sales. Most smokers switched to filter tips because they believed the filters would provide "health protection."

Filter-tipped brands were supposed to reduce the amount of tar and nicotine in smoke that gets sucked directly into the lungs. But in March 1957, Consumers Union tested 33 brands of cigarettes for the nicotine and tar content in their smoke. Test results showed very little difference in the nicotine and tar content of filtered and unfiltered smoke. In 1959, the FTC barred from all ads any mention of filters and tar and nicotine levels.

In 1958, a West Virginia state parks chief reported that filter-tipped cigarettes were turning lake beaches to a tobacco-stain yellow. Cigarettes without filter tips broke down quickly when discarded, but filter tips lasted longer and left a nicotine stain.

Smoking on Campus

From the time of the earliest marketing campaigns, young people have been exposed to cigarette ads. In the 1950s the tobacco companies launched full-scale college promotion programs. In 1959, Philip Morris paid $50 a month to each of 165 campus representatives to hand out free cigarettes. Campus representatives encouraged fraternities to compete with each other in trying to guess football scores correctly. Scores had to be written on the backs of Philip Morris wrappers. Prizes ranged from record

Healthy lung (top)
Cancerous lung (bottom)

In the late 1950s, school principals in Jacksonville, Florida, and the American Cancer Society put on an antismoking educational program in 18 high schools. After the program ended, the pupils' favorite question was "How do I get my parents to quit smoking?"

players and ping-pong tables to trips to Europe. Another contest offered record players in exchange for collected empty cigarette packages. The Liggett & Myers Tobacco Company awarded cars as prizes in its contests.

For years, the main support of college newspapers and magazines had been cigarette advertising. One study showed that cigarette ads accounted for an estimated 40 percent of the advertising incomes of 850 college newspapers. The American Tobacco Company campaigned for college sales by advertising Lucky Strikes in college newspapers and football programs and on campus radio stations. As usual, it gave away free samples. American Tobacco aimed its Tareyton brand directly at college students: "Hooray for college students! They're making Dual Filter Tareyton the big smoke on American campuses! Are you part of this movement? If so, thanks. If not, try 'em!"

In the fall of 1954, Philip Morris decided that a special market like the college market required a "smartly tailored approach." Out of this came the Max Shulman column. In September 1954, humorist Max Shulman started writing "On Campus with Max Shulman." Over 1 million students and numerous college professors read this entertaining column. A line at the bottom of the column read "This column is brought to you by the makers of Philip Morris, who think you would enjoy their cigarette." Some felt that the plan produced the highest readership and sponsor identity of any advertising Philip Morris ever placed.

Capturing a Famous Image

Cigarette advertisers also had a brand new way to pitch cigarettes to college and high school students: plastic-coated book covers that students wrapped around their textbooks. The front covers sported school colors, names, and logos. Back covers carried advertising messages. In 1953, J. P. Lorillard became the first national advertiser to try the back cover. It advertised Old Gold cigarettes.

Other companies changed the target of their products completely in order to gain higher profits. Philip Morris's Marlboro brand was originally marketed as a woman's cigarette with a "Mild as May" slogan. In 1954, Philip Morris hired Leo Burnett, an advertising genius from Chicago. He turned Marlboros from a "feminine" brand into one that appealed to "he-men." Designer Frank Gianninoto created a new package that was red on top and white on the bottom. Moving away from a 30-year tradition, Gianninoto made the Marlboro package a cardboard box with a flip top. When Burnett wanted a tough-guy image for the new Marlboro ads, he decided on cowboys and hired real ones to be his models.

The cowboy Marlboro Man appeared for the first time in January, 1955. For a time, however, the cowboy was only one of many rugged male figures such as football players and race-car drivers used to advertise Marlboros. In 1963, Philip Morris decided to concentrate on the cowboy as the one and only Marlboro Man. Since the 1960s, the sales of Marlboros have continued to climb, making it the number-one-selling cigarette in the world.

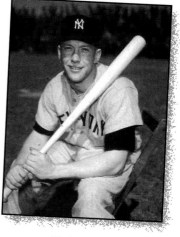

Mickey Mantle

Baseball great Mickey Mantle had appeared in Camel ads in 1955. But by the late 1950s, he was doing ads for Bantron, an anti-smoking pill.

51

CHAPTER SEVEN

A SURGEON GENERAL'S BOMBSHELL

The 1960s was one of the most tumultuous times in United States history. The decade witnessed the assassinations of President John F. Kennedy, his brother Senator Robert F. Kennedy, and civil rights leader, the Reverend Martin Luther King, Jr. The war in Vietnam was broadcast nightly into the homes of millions of Americans. That conflict and racial unrest divided many Americans and made some question the most basic values of our society.

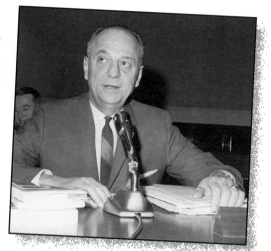

Surgeon General Dr. Luther Terry

In the early 1960s, the Kennedy administration concentrated on fixing problems in the country. Improving people's health was one of the concerns. Health organizations had been pressuring the President (a sometime cigar-smoker) to study the tobacco problem. Kennedy handed the responsibility to Surgeon General Dr. Luther Terry, the nation's leading spokesperson on health issues.

Dr. Terry organized a committee to study the health hazards presented by tobacco. He made sure the tobacco industry had a voice in choosing the committee of experts who studied the problem. That way, tobacco companies could not criticize the findings because they disagreed with the committee's makeup. The committee worked in total secrecy as it reviewed over 7,000 medical articles that dealt with the link between smoking and disease. Hundreds of witnesses were questioned about smoking and health. The tobacco industry supplied key information about the quantities of tobacco smoked annually.

The Surgeon General's report was released at a press conference on Saturday, January 11, 1964. The doors in the press room were locked and no one could leave until the conference ended. Two hundred news reporters received a copy of *Smoking and Health,* the 387-page report. Dr. Terry and his experts then reviewed the whole document for the assembled reporters. After the reporters finished asking questions, they were released to broadcast the news:

"CIGARETTE SMOKING IS A HEALTH HAZARD OF SUFFICIENT IMPORTANCE TO WARRANT APPROPRIATE REMEDIAL ACTION."

The report hit the nation like a bombshell. It became front-page news and a major story on every radio and television station in the United States.

The committee of experts had concluded that smoking causes lung cancer in men, outweighing all other influencing factors including air pollution. Evidence pointed in the same direction for women. The report also stated that cigarette smoking represents a major cause of heart disease, chronic bronchitis, emphysema, and cancer of the larynx. The committee felt filter-tipped cigarettes did little good in preventing disease. The only good news was that smokers could reduce health risks by quitting.

The Surgeon General's report was a landmark. Soon after its release, *The New Yorker* and other magazines stopped taking cigarette advertising.

In 1962, every one of the 20 baseball teams in the expanded Major Leagues had either tobacco or alcohol sponsorship, or both.

A few advertising agencies announced they would no longer do business with cigarette companies. Smokers took antismoking drugs, attended stop-smoking clinics, and bought how-to books on stopping. Many Americans were scared stiff and either cut down on the number of cigarettes they smoked or stopped smoking altogether. As a result, cigarette sales dropped. In 1963, the year before the Surgeon General's report, 523.9 billion cigarettes were sold in the United States. In 1964, the number fell to 511.3 billion.

The FTC Warning
Appears, but Ads Roll On

Shortly after the report was released, the Federal Trade Commission proposed a strong health warning on all cigarette packs and advertisements. The FTC wanted the warnings to mention the risk of death from disease. Congress agreed a warning was need-ed. In 1965, it passed a law with a weaker warning than the kind the FTC wanted. As of January 1, 1966, the Federal Cigarette Labeling and Advertising Act required nine words on all cigarette packages:

"CAUTION: CIGARETTE SMOKING MAY BE HAZARDOUS TO YOUR HEALTH."

In fact, the law was a victory for the tobacco industry because the law temporarily prohibited the FTC and states from requiring health warnings in cigarette advertising. It also prohibited any other health warning on cigarette packs. Not until 1972 did the FTC get more of what it wanted. Then

In 1964, teens aged 14 through 18 attended the National Conference on Smoking and Youth. The federal government set up the conference to get reactions from young people on the issue of smoking and youth.

How effective are restrictions in preventing smoking? Many felt that the acceptance of regulations depended on their enforcement. Rules that are easily broken are not respected.

The delegates suggested that a massive educational effort was required to enlighten the public about smoking and health. How do you make nonsmoking respectable and acceptable? Use the motivational appeals of advertising in reverse by using pictures and testimonials of non-smokers who are admired by youth. (This is particularly effec-tive for children or preteens.)

Indirect methods are judged more effective than the more direct "Don't smoke, it will kill you." Most youth agreed that the slogan or joke will be remembered longer.

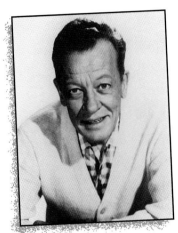

William Talman

William Talman, the actor who played the prosecutor on *Perry Mason*, the popular television show that ran from 1957 to 1965, filmed an antismoking commercial in July 1968. He was dying of lung cancer and had only a few weeks to live. He said: "You know, I didn't really mind losing the courtroom battles. But I'm in a battle right now I don't want to lose at all . . . I've got lung cancer. So take some advice about smoking and losing from someone who's been doing both for years. If you haven't smoked—don't start. If you do smoke—quit. Don't be a loser." In great pain, Talman managed one smile during the commercial. He died August 30, 1968.

cigarette ads were required to include health warnings.

The tobacco industry feared more government regulation, so it promised to police itself. In January 1964 the tobacco industry itself established the Cigarette Advertising Code. The industry promised to stop pitching ads to young people under the age of 21. That meant no more advertising in college publications, comic books, and newspaper sections with comics. It promised to drop testimonials by famous athletes. It also promised to stop claiming that smoking improved health, glamour, and social life. It promised to use models who were at least 25 years old. Four months after the code was written, Viceroy ads showed young tennis players lighting up after a game. The models might have been 25 years old, but some didn't look it. One TV commercial producer admitted he had tried to find older models who "looked young."

After the code went into effect, cigarette advertisers were not supposed to advertise on TV programs with a large number of viewers under 21. Nevertheless, cigarette advertisers sponsored *The Twilight Zone, Wide World of Sports, The Beverly Hillbillies* and many other programs with large youth audiences. Children and teenagers were exposed to hundreds of seductive cigarette messages. In a typical week in 1966, tobacco companies spent about $3 million to air 3,000 commercials urging viewers to smoke 38 different brands!

A Watchful Young Viewer

Tobacco companies had other ways to promote their brands on television. They helped support professional sports teams. In 1963, R. J. Reynolds sponsored eight different baseball teams, and the American Tobacco Company sponsored six.

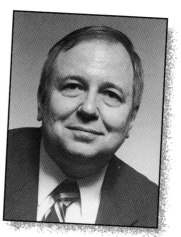

John F. Banzhaf III

Philip Morris sponsored National Football League games on CBS, Brown & Williamson sponsored college football bowl games, and J. P. Lorillard was a sponsor of the 1964 Olympics.

On Thanksgiving Day, 1966, John F. Banzhaf III, a young lawyer, was watching a cigarette-sponsored football game. When the network interrupted the game several times with cigarette commercials, Banzhaf became outraged. He knew cigarette smoking was controversial and that commercials only gave the pro-smoking point of view. He knew about the "fairness doctrine" of the Federal Communications Commission (FCC) that required recipients of broadcast licenses to present all sides of controversial subjects. Banzhaf filed a complaint with the FCC, asking it to apply the fairness doctrine to cigarette commercials. To the surprise of all, it did. The FCC required all radio and television stations broadcasting cigarette commercials to donate "significant" free airtime for antismoking messages.

In February of 1968, John F. Banzhaf III, the man responsible for the FCC ruling, quit law and formed Action on Smoking and Health (ASH), a new antismoking organization. Banzhaf declared ASH "both a nickname and a goal—the end of cigarettes." ASH is a national nonprofit legal action and educational organization that fights for the rights of nonsmokers. It uses the power of the law to represent nonsmokers in courts and legislative bodies and before regulatory agencies. It publishes a quarterly newsletter, *ASH Smoking and Health Report.*

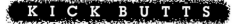

In 1969, the U.S. Public Health Service gave teens in Bakersfield, California, a grant of $47,000 to see if they could get antismoking messages across to teens more effectively than adults could. The high school students set up their own advertising agency and created "Smoke Out," an antismoking ad campaign. First, the teens surveyed the smoking habits of students in three Bakersfield schools. Then they asked ad agency professionals for information on planning and running the campaign.

The student ad agency decided to make smoking look insulting by using bumper stickers ("Smoke . . Choke . . Croak!"), posters, billboard messages, buttons, book covers, and newspaper public service ads all produced by the Smoke Out crew. One TV spot showed a shot of an elegantly dressed woman. "She smokes." Shot of burning trash. "So does the city dump."

The tobacco industry, congressional representatives from tobacco-growing states, and the broadcasters expressed shock. The FCC rejected the petitions of the tobacco industry and the broadcasters to do away with its fairness doctrine order. It reaffirmed its ruling requiring free time for antismoking messages over the objections of tobacco companies and broadcasters. Lee Loevinger, FCC commissioner, declared that "suggesting cigarette smoking to young people, in the light of present-day knowledge, is something very close to wickedness."

As a result of the FCC ruling, many health agencies and the U.S. Public Health Service produced TV and radio spots condemning smoking. One message showed a young person puffing and coughing in a bathroom. Then a voice was heard saying: "Remember your first cigarette? Maybe your body was trying to tell you something?" Between July 1, 1967, and December 31, 1970, these and other antismoking messages were aired at no cost on television alongside paid commercials promoting cigarette smoking. The results? Although the tobacco industry was spending over $200 million a year to promote cigarettes, cigarette consumption declined. A survey of teenagers exposed to antismoking messages showed a sharp decrease in the number of teenagers taking up cigarettes.

Finally, the FCC recommended to Congress that all cigarette ads be banned from TV and radio. In March 1970, Congress outlawed cigarette ads on TV and radio. The law also strengthened the health warning on cigarette packs (but not on smokeless tobacco products). The warning read as follows:

WARNING: THE SURGEON GENERAL HAS DETERMINED THAT CIGARETTE SMOKING IS DANGEROUS TO YOUR HEALTH.

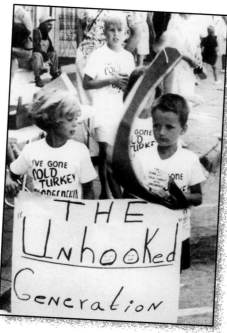

Going "cold turkey" in Iowa

The law became effective on January 2, 1971, four years, one month, and nine days after the Thanksgiving Day telecast that prompted John Banzhaf III to take action against cigarette advertising.

In 1969, the town of Greenfield, Iowa, went "cold turkey." Some 376 smokers threw their cartons of cigarettes into a bonfire and signed no-smoking pledges. The town was helping to promote *Cold Turkey*, a movie being filmed in Greenfield about a millionaire who promises a fictional town $25 million if all the residents stop smoking. In real life, United Artists promised the town $6,000 if smokers signed a pledge to quit puffing for 30 days. At the end of the month, merchants reported that cigarette sales had decreased by 30 percent. And 134 townsfolk claimed to have gone the full 30 days without smoking.

CHAPTER EIGHT

THE SMOKE-FREE MOVEMENT BLOSSOMS

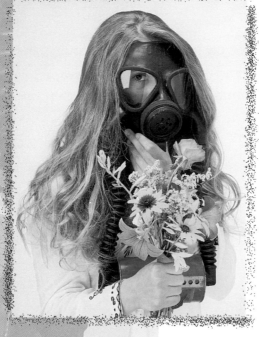

During the years that TV showed thousands of antismoking messages, smoking rates dropped. In 1967, 549.3 billion cigarettes were consumed. In 1968, 545.6 billion cigarettes were consumed. In 1969, 528.9 billion were smoked. Government statistics showed that as many as 10 million Americans quit smoking from 1967 to 1970.

Antismoking groups felt their public-service announcements were successful. They also felt that tobacco companies knew the messages stopped people from smoking. In 1971, when cigarette advertising disappeared from TV, so did the antismoking commercials. Broadcasters no longer were required to give "significant amounts" of free airtime for the antismoking messages. Without constant reminders of how bad smoking was for their health, Americans resumed their old habits. In 1971, cigarette use bounced back, to 555.1 billion cigarettes smoked annually.

After the TV and radio ban, where did all the cigarette advertising go? Tobacco companies poured hundreds of millions of advertising dollars into newspapers, magazines, and billboards. For example, from January 5 to 7, 1970, the *Chicago Tribune* carried 65-column inches (that's how newspapers measure space) of cigarette ads. A year later, it carried 170-column inches of cigarette advertising. *The Washington Post* published 56-column inches in 1970 and 119-column inches in 1971. In 1970, before the TV and radio ban, tobacco companies spent

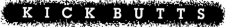

In April of 1970, a smoking with-drawal clinic, teenage-style, was held for a week at Dallastown Area High school in York County, Pennsylvania, the heart of the state's handmade-cigar country. The school nurse and the princi-pal, along with local health agen-cies, set up the program. The principal and the faculty selected 45 students whose records showed that they were heavy smokers. They ranged in age from 13 to 18.

On the first day of the clinic, a physician talked to the teens about withdrawal symptoms. Then the adults stepped aside. The stu-dents divided themselves into six teams and chose their own team leaders. At the end of the 5-day clinic, a total of 34 cigarettes were smoked in a day, down from 709 cigarettes smoked the day before the clinic began.

$14 million on newspaper advertising. In 1979, the figure rose to almost $241 million.

Luring More Women Into the Habit

Tobacco companies shifted their advertising efforts to attract more women. For decades, the cigarette industry had done everything it could to attract women to smoking, from hiring movie stars to using stylish-looking young models to appear in ads. In 1968, Philip Morris put out Virginia Slims, a cigarette strictly for women. The Virginia Slims' slogan, "You've come a long way, baby," appealed to women who wanted to do as they pleased.

In the 1970s, advertising for Virginia Slims and other cigarette brands flooded women's magazines, newspapers, and Sunday supplements. By 1979, cigarettes were the most advertised product in some women's magazines, with as many as 20 ads in a single issue. The tobacco industry admitted that it targeted stressed-out working women as the ideal candidates for cigarettes.

After cigarette companies targeted their adver-tising to women, the numbers of women smokers grew at a faster rate. But women were not the only ones who saw these ads. Girls saw them, too, and were swept away by the glamorous images of energetic joggers, bikers, and backpackers appearing in the ads. By 1971, the numbers of girls smoking at 13, 14, and 15 increased. In 1979, surveys showed more girls smoked than boys.

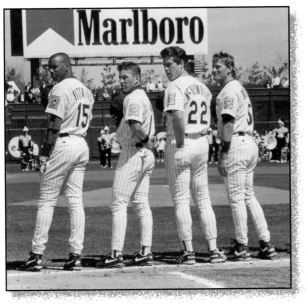

Cigarette advertising at Shea Stadium

Promotions helped enrich the tobacco companies. In 1971, the same year that federal law banned cigarette ads from television and radio, Philip Morris launched a series of tennis matches called the Virginia Slims Invitational. Also in 1971, Winston Cup auto racing began. TV cameras showed cigarette logos on stock cars and stadium billboards with tobacco ads. Sporting events put cigarettes back on television, even though there was a law banning cigarette advertising on TV.

Secondhand Smoke

Until the mid-1970s, concern about tobacco was limited to how smoking harmed smokers. But when people became concerned about air pollution from cars, incinerators, and power plants, they began to

In November 1970, there were 737 students from Oklahoma City high schools who were studied by physicians to see if cigarette smoking had any effects on their lungs. The medical survey showed that students who smoked cigarettes had far more respiratory symptoms than those who did not smoke.

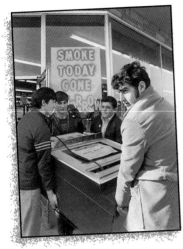

1977 Smokeout Drive

In 1974, the Great American Smokeout began with Lynn Smith, publisher of the *Monticello* (MN) *Times*. Smith suggested that the townspeople try to quit smoking for a day. Three months later, 10 percent of the 300 people who quit had succeeded in staying tobacco-free. That year, the event went statewide. In 1977, the American Cancer Society launched the Great American Smokeout as a national event, held annually on the third Thursday in November.

worry about secondhand smoke from cigarettes. Nonsmokers argued that cigarette smoke smelled bad, irritated their eyes, burned their noses, and gave them headaches. People with allergies were bothered by cigarette smoke. In 1976, the New Jersey Superior Court ruled that a Clifton, New Jersey, office worker allergic to tobacco smoke had the right to work in a smoke-free office.

Nonsmokers were beginning to demand separate smoking and no-smoking sections in restaurants, airplanes, buses, trains, and other public places. In 1975, legislators from both political parties in Minnesota passed a Clean Indoor Air Act. It was aimed at protecting the quality of indoor air, not at punishing smokers. It provided no-smoking areas in all public buildings and soon became the model for other states. In 1980, a *Minneapolis Tribune* public opinion poll found that 92 percent of nonsmokers and 87 percent of heavy smokers favored the law.

A National Bill of Rights for the Nonsmoker

During the 1970s, very little was known about the effects of secondhand smoke on nonsmokers. Scientists were not ready to say for certain that exposure to tobacco smoke caused serious illness in nonsmokers. The medical community and health groups did not focus on "passive smoking," as the issue became known. This came later. But Surgeon General Jesse Steinfeld paid attention to passive smoking. In November 1971, he called for

In 1976, filmmaker Peter Taylor interviewed six real-life American cowboys for his 27-minute documentary titled *Death in the West*. Taylor contrasted the macho image of the Marlboro Man with the lives of the six cowboys. All were heavy smokers at one time. All were dying from lung cancer or emphysema.

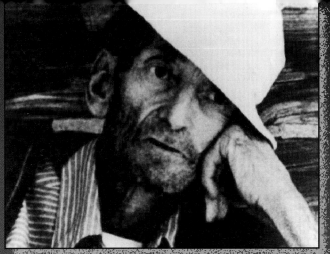

Shortly after *Death in the West* was shown on British television, the American Cancer Society and CBS-TV's *60 Minutes* expressed interest in the American broadcast rights to the film. Philip Morris went to court in London, England, to prevent Thames Television from selling the film or showing it again.

Thames and Philip Morris settled out of court and all copies of the film except one (it was locked in Thames's vault) were handed over to Philip Morris. On December 1, 1981, Dr. Stanton Glantz, an associate professor at the University of California at San Francisco, received a copy of *Death in the West*. Five months later, the film was back on TV, this time in San Francisco. By the time the film was shown in the United States, five of the six cowboys had died.

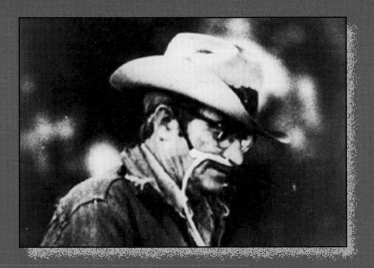

a national bill of rights for the nonsmoker. He wanted bans on smoking in public places such as restaurants, public transportation, and theaters. Steinfeld received thousands of letters in support of smoke-free air.

The tobacco industry was worried about the emerging nonsmokers' rights movement. In 1978, the Roper Organization conducted a secret study for the tobacco industry. The study concluded the following:

1. A majority of Americans believed it was probably hazardous to be around people who smoke, even if they are not smoking themselves.

2. A steadily increasing majority of Americans believe that the tobacco industry knows that the case against cigarettes is true.

3. More than nine out of ten Americans believed that smoking was hazardous to a smoker's health.

4. A majority of people wanted separate smoking sections in public places.

Then, the Roper study concluded with a statement that really rattled the tobacco industry: "What the smoker does to himself may be his business, but what the smoker does to the non-smoker is quite a different matter. . . ."

This was a remarkable statement because there was not much evidence in 1978 that passive smoking did long-term damage to nonsmokers.

BARFBORO BARFING TEAM

In 1977, Doctors Ought To Care (DOC) was founded in Miami, Florida, by Dr. Alan Blum. He got the idea for the organization when he spoke at a drug treatment center where most of the teens were smoking cigarettes. By the end of his talk, in which he had made fun of ads in the teen magazines, he noticed that everyone had put out their cigarettes.

DOC, now an international organization of health professionals, is located in Houston, Texas. Years ago, it launched a national counteradvertising campaign to offset the promotion of what it calls lethal lifestyles, especially tobacco advertising. DOC ran a Dead Man Chew Softball Tournament, an Emphysema Slims Celebrity Tennis Tournament, and a Smoke-free Jazz Fest. In 1993, DOC wanted to undermine the Marlboro Adventure team's U.S. debut. It repainted a Volkswagen van, calling it a Barfmobile. It

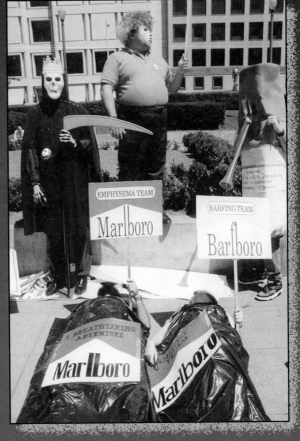

Barfboro Demonstration

printed thousands of Barfboro Barf Bags—in red and white—and created the Barfboro Barfing team. In 1994 the Barfing team coordinated dozens of community activities designed to get young people to laugh at the Marlboro Adventure team. The team sells a "Barfboro" line of items including lunch bags, posters, T-shirts, stickers, and pins.

It sells "Virginia Slime" and "New Corpse" posters as well as a "Throw-Tobacco-Out-of-Sports Cardboard Boomerang" and videos. DOC's *Journal of Medical Activism* covers activities.

CHAPTER NINE

SMOKE-FREE RIGHTS ARE HERE TO STAY

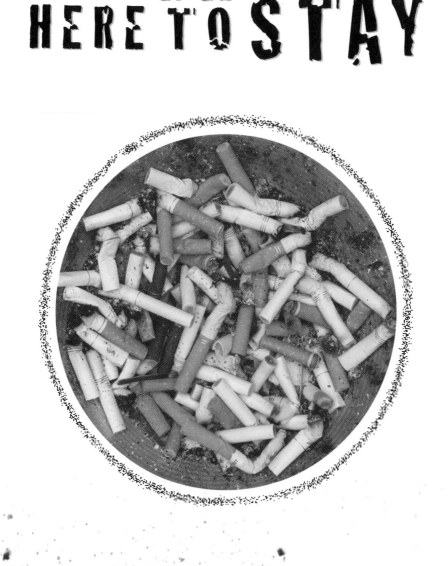

The 1980s began with a troubled economy. It wasn't as bad as the Great Depression of the 1930s, but it was still bad enough for many thousands of people. By the end of 1982, ten million Americans were out of work.

The Health Conscience of the Nation

The President during most of the 1980s was Ronald Reagan. He appointed C. Everett Koop, a family doctor, as Surgeon General because he thought Koop shared his conservative values of less government involvement in the lives of Americans. As it turned out, Koop valued public health more than conservatism. He spoke his mind and, as a result, became the health conscience of the nation.

While Surgeon General Koop was in office, seven reports on the health hazards of smoking were released. In February 1982, Koop's office released a report on cancer, which turned out be one of the strongest antismoking reports the U.S. Public Health Service had ever produced. According to the report, 85 percent of the lung cancer deaths would not have happened if the victims had never smoked. At the press conference where the report was released, Koop said: "Cigarette smoking is the chief preventable cause of death in our society." He would repeat this statement countless times afterward.

The next three years brought more hard-hitting reports from the Surgeon General. The 1983

In 1980, the American Council on Science and Health (ACSH) did the first of several surveys of popular magazines. (ACSH is a consumer-education group located in New York City. It was founded in 1978 and publishes *Priorities,* a journal that discusses issues related to food, drugs, chemicals, lifestyle, the environment, and health.) In its 1982 survey, for example, it looked at 18 large-circulation magazines that discussed health issues during the period from 1965 to 1981. The survey found that the best coverage of tobacco/health issues was in magazines that did not accept cigarette ads. Among the best magazines covering smoking and health were *Reader's Digest, Prevention,* and *Seventeen.* The worst coverage was found in *Ms., Newsweek,* and *Parade.*

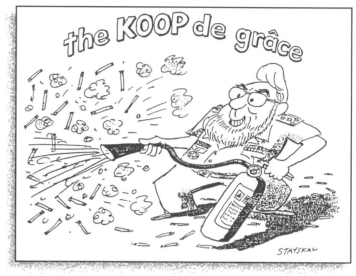

Surgeon General Koop in action

In 1984, Olympic diving champion Greg Louganis wanted to be the national chairman of the Great American Smokeout sponsored by the American Cancer Society. He couldn't do it. Years later he explained why: "My success at diving made me a role model for children, but I was pressured to avoid national exposure of what I knew about smoking because it was against the interests of Philip Morris (the company that owned the California facility where he trained). With the Olympics only a few months away, I had no choice but to turn down the chairmanship. . . . By sponsoring sporting events and facilities, tobacco companies made athletes and sports associations indebted to and dependent upon them."

report dealt with the connection between cigarette smoking and heart disease. The 1984 report dealt with the connection between cigarette smoking and chronic bronchitis and emphysema. In 1985, Koop's report pointed out that for American workers, cigarette smoking represented a greater cause of death and disability than their workplace environment.

The Proof

By 1986, smoke-free supporters wanted to pass more laws to protect nonsmokers in the workplace and public places. But they needed proof that secondhand smoke endangered nonsmokers. Koop's 1986 report delivered that proof. It said "involuntary smoking is a cause of disease, including lung cancer, in healthy nonsmokers." It especially stressed the harmful effects of passive smoking in public places and workplaces. It concluded that simple separation of smokers and nonsmokers within the same air-space reduces but does not eliminate exposure to environmental tobacco smoke.

More doctors and scientists released other studies during the decade. All linked secondhand smoke to lung cancer. The evidence was mounting and helped support the demand for smoke-free environments. Congress acted and banned smoking aboard all domestic airline flights of two hours or less. Dr. Everett R. Rhoades, director of the Indian Health Service (IHS), banned all indoor smoking in IHS clinics, hospitals, and offices nationwide. Following that move, the Department of Health and Human Services established a smoke-free environment in all of its buildings. In 1987, voters in Greensboro, North Carolina—the heart of tobacco country—approved a tough local smoking law in spite of heavy opposition by tobacco companies. In February 1988 the International Olympic Committee banned smoking in Olympic villages, on public transportation, in arenas, and in some restaurants. Also in 1988 the Democrats made history in Atlanta, Georgia, when they held the first smoke-free national political convention in U. S. history.

In 50 years of *Superman* comics, Lois Lane never smoked. Then Philip Morris paid $42,500 to feature Marlboro ads in the movie *Superman II*. Suddenly, Lois Lane began chain-smoking Marlboro Lights.

The War on Smokeless Tobacco

Koop was a busy Surgeon General. Besides turning out the report on passive smoking, he targeted smokeless tobacco: chewing, or spit tobacco, and snuff. Smokeless tobacco products had become

"DON'T DIP SNUFF."

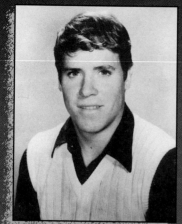

On February 25, 1984, Sean Marsee, a 19-year-old Oklahoma high school track star, died from mouth cancer. Sean had been a terrific athlete. He took care of himself and didn't smoke or drink. He lifted weights, watched his diet, ran five miles a day six months of the year. He won 28 medals running the anchor leg on the 400-meter relay. He was voted Talihina High's outstanding athlete for 1983.

There was one thing Sean did that he believed was safe. Since 1977, when he was twelve years old, he had been dipping snuff. A tobacco company had handed him free samples at a rodeo near his home in Oklahoma. Five years later, Sean developed cancer of the mouth. He was stunned. Sean's coach did not make a big deal about dipping. And snuff was advertised on television.

In 1983, part of Sean's tongue was removed. During his second operation, he had radical neck surgery. His third operation cost him his jawbone. But none of the operations stopped the cancer from spreading. Before Sean died, a friend asked him if he would like to share something about his ordeal with young athletes. He penciled (he could no longer talk) "Don't dip snuff."

A year after Sean died, his mother filed a suit against the United States Tobacco Company, manufacturer of *Copenhagen Snuff*, the brand Sean used. She asked for millions of dollars in punitive damages. Expert medical testimony linked smokeless tobacco with oral cancer. The tobacco company said there was no evidence proving its products caused cancer. The jury agreed with the tobacco company.

Two years after Sean Marsee died, Congress passed a law requiring the rotation of three warning labels on smokeless tobacco products and advertisements.

WARNING: This Product May Cause Mouth Cancer

WARNING: This Product May Cause Gum Disease and Result in Tooth Loss

WARNING: This Product Is Not a Safe Alternative to Cigarette Smoking

The law also stopped the advertising of smokeless tobacco on TV and radio.

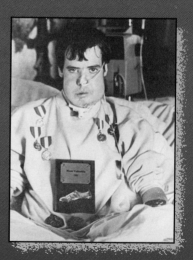

popular again for the first time since the late 1800s and early 1900s. While cigarette smoking was declining, the use of snuff was rising among teenagers and young men. Between 1970 and 1985, moist-snuff use increased by 30 percent among all Americans, but eightfold in the 17- to 19-year-old groups. A large part of the rise was the result of heavy advertising.

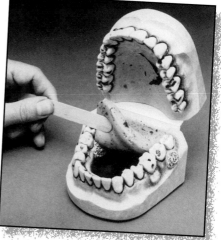

The United States Tobacco Company (UST), maker of SKOAL and Copenhagen, displayed its products alongside candy in neighborhood grocery stores, gas stations, and truck stops across the nation. In 1983 the same company introduced SKOAL Bandits, an easy-to-use tea bag of snuff. Its slogan, "Take a pouch instead of a puff," attracted teens. Doctors have called the pouch "a low nicotine teaching tool" that allows beginners to slowly develop a "taste" for snuff. Once addicted to snuff, "dippers" move on to the more addictive brands.

Smokeless tobacco companies market their products in a variety of ways. Besides advertising on billboards and in sports magazines, UST has hired famous football players to promote SKOAL in personal appearances. The smokeless tobacco companies leave no avenue unexplored in selling their products. They sponsor sports and cultural events such as softball games, rodeos, drag races, tractor pulls, and country music concerts.

Another powerful marketing tool is the free sample. Major league pitcher Nolan Ryan has said that smoking cigarettes and chewing tobacco

In 1985, STAT (Stop Teenage Addiction to Tobacco) in Springfield, Massachusetts, was founded as a nonprofit corporation to focus on reducing the use of tobacco by children and teens. STAT community organizers and trainers support tobacco control and fight advertising efforts by the tobacco companies, especially ads and promotions aimed at children and teens. Teens worked at STAT headquarters, took part in its annual conference, and helped in community projects. It published the *Tobacco-Free Youth Reporter*.

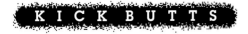

In January 1986, Americans for Nonsmokers' Rights (ANR) was organized. It is a national anti-smoking organization devoted to clean indoor air legislation and nonsmokers' rights. ANR has assisted in the passage of scores of city and county clean indoor air ordinances. It publishes *ANR Update,* a quarterly newsletter that carries the latest news and developments in nonsmokers' rights.

In 1987, ANR launched its "Teens as Teachers" project. It trains high school students to help teach younger children in elementary school, using ANR's "Death in the West" and "Second-hand Smoke" programs. These programs use nonsmokers and a group of teens who have stopped smoking as teachers. Teen teachers address addiction versus free choice, the right to smoke-free air, how to pick apart glamorous cigarette ads, and how kids can protect themselves from second-hand smoke.

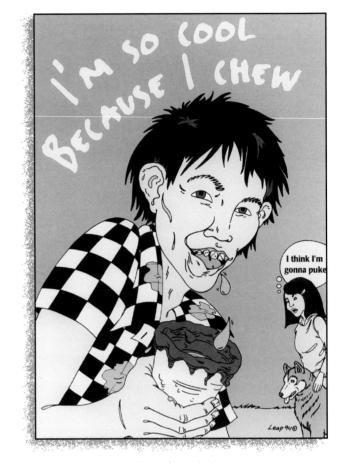

Poster from Alaska

declined among baseball players during the 1980s, but dipping snuff increased. "The switch came with free samples of dip coming into the clubhouse," Ryan said. Players have served as unpaid models for tobacco companies, too. Most importantly, close-up television shots of star baseball players chewing or using dip have been seen by millions of young people.

Surgeon General Koop was alarmed by the health hazards of smokeless tobacco. He took action by appointing a committee to study the

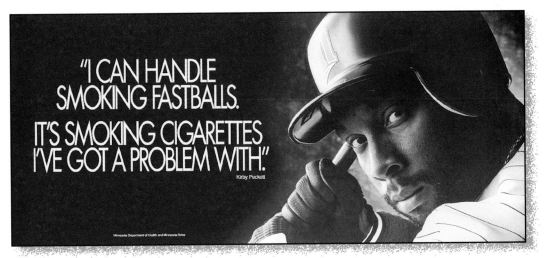

Kirby Puckett antitobacco poster

problem. The committee concluded with these strong words: "The oral use of smokeless tobacco represents a significant health risk. It is not a safe substitute for smoking cigarettes. It can cause cancer . . . and lead to nicotine addiction."

After Koop's report on smokeless tobacco was released, major league baseball worked with the National Cancer Institute to develop a guide to help major and minor league players quit using smokeless tobacco. The Los Angeles Dodgers went even further. The team banned all its players from carrying snuff or chew while in uniform.

Historic Health Warnings

After Koop's committee produced the report on smokeless tobacco, the Surgeon General turned his attention to nicotine addiction. Here was the heart of the issue. The Surgeon General's 1988 report

In 1987, the American Lung Association conducted a telephone survey called "Teens Prefer to Date Nonsmokers." The question posed was: Do you prefer to date a smoker or a nonsmoker? Seventy-eight percent of the boys ages 12 to 17 and 69 percent of the girls in that age range said they preferred to date nonsmokers. One percent of the teens questioned said they preferred to date a smoker.

CANCER COUNTRY

Melissa Antonow, a fifth grader in New York City, drew a winning poster that appeared in every subway car in New York. Melissa's poster—"Come to where the Cancer is"—was part of the first prohealth ad contest for New York City schoolchildren run by Joe Cherner's SmokeFree Educational Services. Cherner's group, founded in 1987, educates people about the benefits of being tobacco-free and the unhealthy consequences of breathing secondhand smoke. The contest Melissa took part in received national and world attention. A publisher printed 46 full-color posters by the students who entered the Smoke-Free Ad contest.

Cherner, who draws no salary, has created parodies of cigarette ads that have appeared on New York City cabs since early 1997. Having pledged to use his early success on Wall Street to do good, he continues his fight against tobacco.

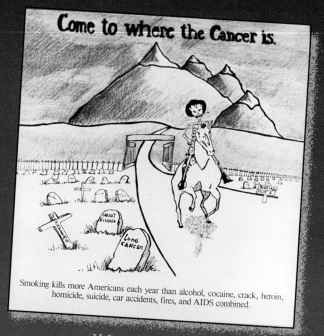

Smoking kills more Americans each year than alcohol, cocaine, crack, heroin, homicide, suicide, car accidents, fires, and AIDS combined.

Melissa Antonow's poster

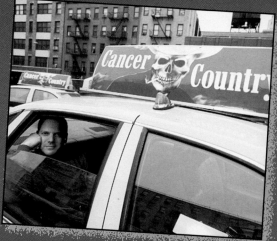

Joe Cherner

branded nicotine as a highly addictive substance. Like heroin and cocaine, the addictive qualities of nicotine make the smoker physically crave tobacco. It is hard to quit nicotine. For some users, it takes an average of five attempts to give up the habit. Koop wanted cigarettes to carry a warning label that read as follows: "Surgeon General's Warning: Tobacco Contains Nicotine, an Addictive Drug."

The tobacco companies fought hard against any labels, and Koop did not get the warning he wanted. But the companies agreed to add four warning labels to cigarette packs and ads as a way of avoiding the addiction warning. On October 12, 1984, President Ronald Reagan signed the Comprehensive Smoking Education Act. It replaced the previous health warning on cigarette packages and ads with four rotating strongly worded health warnings

1. SURGEON GENERAL'S WARNING: Smoking Causes Lung Cancer, Heart Disease, Emphysema, and May Complicate Pregnancy.

2. SURGEON GENERAL'S WARNING: Quitting Smoking Now Greatly Reduces Serious Risks to Your Health.

3. SURGEON GENERAL'S WARNING: Smoking by Pregnant Women May Result in Fetal Injury, Premature Birth, and Low Birth Weight.

4. SURGEON GENERAL'S WARNING: Cigarette Smoke Contains Carbon Monoxide.

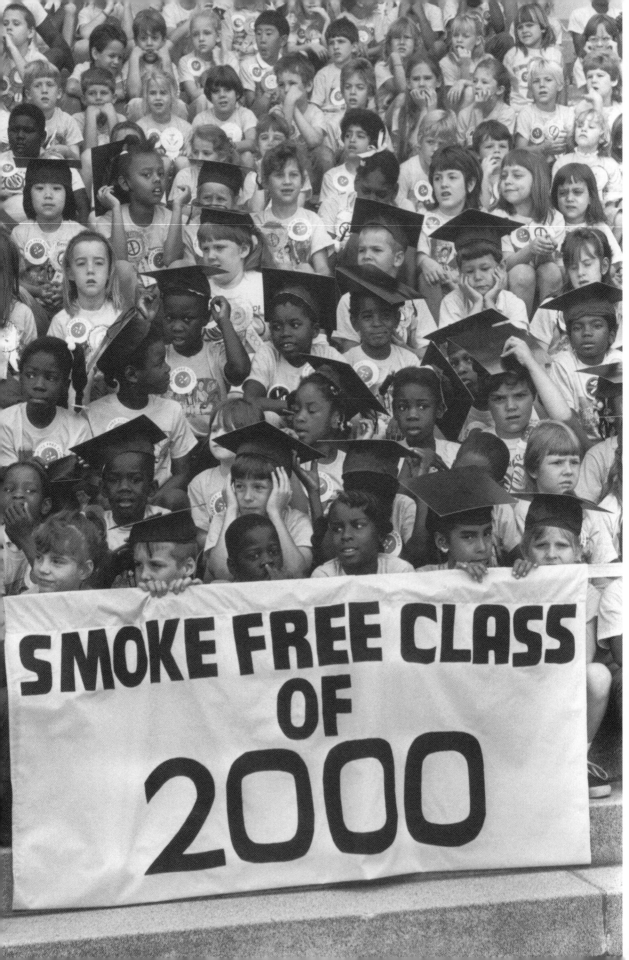

SMOKE FREE CLASS OF 2000

The warnings took effect one year later. The Smoking Education Act also required cigarette companies to disclose all chemicals and other ingredients added to cigarettes during the manufacturing process. In addition, the act created a federal Office on Smoking and Health and a new federal council to coordinate and oversee federal, private, and research efforts concerning the health hazards of smoking.

In 1989, Koop released his final report. It highlighted the important gains made in preventing smoking-related diseases. While C. Everett Koop was Surgeon General, smoking rates in the United States dropped from 33 percent to 26 percent of the population. Koop felt that his reports on passive smoking and addiction hit the tobacco companies where they could feel it. The report on passive smoking showed smoke that comes off the burning end of cigarettes hurts nonsmokers. The addiction report showed smoking was not a matter of free choice for smokers because nicotine made smoking a physical necessity.

To sum up his efforts, Koop boldly called for a smoke-free society by the year 2000. He wanted teachers, doctors, the media, and government to ensure that the high school graduating class of the year 2000 was smoke-free.

Another target of Koop's crusade was cigarette advertising. It angered him that cigarette ads, although banned from television, had sneaked back on TV through sports events sponsored by tobacco

A group of health agencies rallied to Surgeon General Koop's call to create a smoke-free society by the year 2000. They created the "Smoke-Free Class of 2000" program. The curriculum kicked off in 1988 when about 1 million first graders learned about the health hazards of smoking. The program aims to help students remain tobacco-free when they graduate from high school. To accomplish this, the youngsters receive antismoking messages throughout each of their school years. At the junior and senior high levels, students take action in the community. One of the Surgeon General's granddaughters—a first grader in 1988—will be among the smoke-free class of 2000.

companies. Motor racing became one of the major promotional activities used by the tobacco industry. Through its Winston and Camel brands, the R. J. Reynolds Tobacco Company was the leading sponsor of automobile and motorcycle racing in the United States. Philip Morris also sponsored motor racing. When viewers watched a race, they saw officials wearing the Marlboro logo on their clothing, and cars and drivers sporting the Marlboro name.

Kids in low-income neighborhoods see more billboards with tobacco ads than kids in higher-income neighborhoods do. A 1986 Department of Planning survey in San Francisco, California, found that 62 percent of the billboards in African American neighborhoods

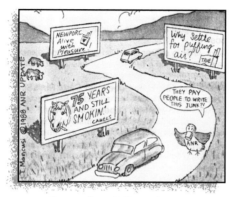

Cartoon from ANR Update *targets billboards*

and 42 percent in Latino neighborhoods advertised cigarettes and alcoholic drinks compared to only 36 percent of the billboards advertising those citywide. A 1987 study in St. Louis, Missouri, found that there were four times more tobacco and alcohol ads in that city's African American neighborhoods than in its white neighborhoods.

Koop was especially disturbed that ads targeted young people, women, and minorities through magazines, promotions, and billboards. Billboard ads associated smoking with financial success, robust activity, athletics, social acceptance, romance, glamour, healthy outdoor fun, and even good health. Interestingly, the ads showed well-off people smoking—yet, in reality, higher-income groups were smoking less.

Whose Freedom?

There was also the issue of freedom. Koop was angered when tobacco companies talked about free choice and free speech but actually encouraged addiction. In Koop's words, "Nicotine addicts do not enjoy free choice." In the Surgeon General's view, tobacco companies were "great enemies of freedom" who "use their economic clout [power] to force publishers not to print articles about the real consequences of smoking." Finally, Koop and others criticized the American tobacco industry for promoting cigarette use among women and children in Asia, Africa, and South America, new markets where the harmful effects of cigarette smoking were not known. For example, in the 1980s the U.S. government pressured Japan to suspend taxes on U.S. cigarettes. As a result, the Japanese market was opened. Japanese men were already heavy smokers. The new market consisted of women and young people. Smoking among Japanese women rose from 8.6 percent in 1986 to 18.2 percent in 1991. The same strategies were applied in other countries.

In June 1988, a Newark, New Jersey, court ruled that cigarette manufacturers were liable for the death of a smoker. It was the first time in history that such a ruling had been handed down. The court awarded $400,000 to the husband of Rose Cipollone, who died of lung cancer in 1984 at the age of 58. Rose had been a heavy smoker throughout her life. In January 1990 the verdict was reversed by the Third Circuit Court of Appeals in Philadelphia. The case went to the U.S. Supreme Court, which handed down a landmark decision in June 1992. The Supreme Court ruled that the warning label on cigarette packs did not shield tobacco makers from being liable for damages. The decision cleared the way for lawsuits accusing tobacco companies of deceiving the public about the health hazards of smoking. The Cipollone case was sent back to the district court in New Jersey for a retrial, but the Cipollone family dropped the appeal.

CHAPTER TEN

THE WAR ON TOBACCO IN THE 1990s

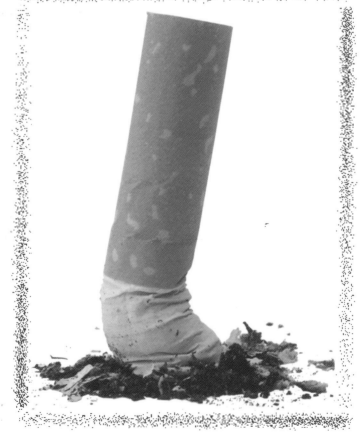

In the 1990s, people voted for change. When President George Bush ran for reelection in 1992, he lost to William Jefferson Clinton, who made reforming the nation's health care system a top goal. Soon after taking office, President Clinton appointed his wife, Hillary Rodham Clinton, to head a committee on health care. The committee proposed guaranteeing all Americans a minimum package of benefits. Congress, however, did not move on the proposal.

The Focus on Tobacco Sharpens

Health care reform ground to a halt during Clinton's first term, but health care costs continued to rise. A major factor driving up health care costs is tobacco abuse and the serious illnesses resulting from smoking and secondhand smoke. Catastrophic illnesses such as lung cancer, bronchitis, emphysema, asthma, and heart disease cost people a fortune in doctor and hospital bills. According to Joseph Califano, former Secretary of Health, Education, and Welfare, smoking is the largest single drain on Medicare, a national health insurance program for 37 million people.

Both Clintons understand the terrible toll that cigarettes take on the nation's health and have spoken out against smoking. Neither the President nor the First Lady smokes cigarettes. President Clinton smokes cigars on rare occasions, however. The White House is a smoke-free presidential home. As parents of a teenage daughter, the Clintons are well aware of the allure that cigarettes

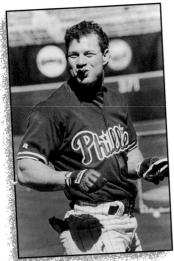

Lenny Dykstra no longer chews tobacco.

On March 7, 1991, Baseball Commissioner Fay Vincent announced that the use of smokeless tobacco would be forbidden in four rookie and Class A minor leagues, the levels at which most young men enter professional baseball. After the ban went into effect in 1993, Travis Baptist of the Class AA Minor League Knoxville Smokies was ejected from a game for chewing tobacco in the dugout.

have for young people. The president listened to David Kessler—a pediatrician with a law degree and the commissioner of the Food and Drug Administration (FDA)—testify about the addictive qualities of tobacco. Kessler pointed out that "a person who hasn't started smoking by age 19 is unlikely to ever become a smoker. Nicotine addiction begins when most tobacco users are teenagers, so let's call this what it really is: a pediatric disease." Dr. Kessler called for cigarette regulation and a wide-reaching program to prevent youngsters from becoming addicted to nicotine.

Smoke-Free Youth: A National Priority

President Clinton agreed that a program geared to youth was needed and that the federal government should deliver that program. In August 1995, Clinton announced a plan to combat smoking among children and teenagers. In the President's words, "Less smoking means less cancer, less illness, longer lives, [and] a stronger America." One of the first steps in Clinton's plan was to grant the FDA the power to curb cigarette marketing and sales. His aim was to reduce tobacco use by children and teenagers under 18 by 50 percent in seven years. This was the first time in the nation's history that a President made preventing tobacco use among youth a national priority.

Creating a smoke-free society won't be easy, however. The FDA will have a tough time regulating the tobacco industry. The roadblocks include

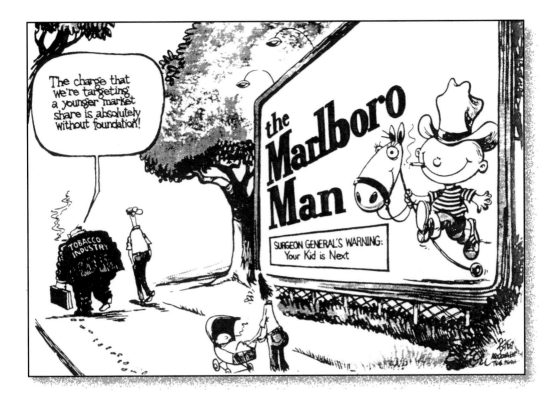

lawmakers from tobacco-producing states—who oppose regulation of the tobacco industry—and the tobacco industry itself. Vending-machine owners have not approved government regulation, either. Advertisers of tobacco products argue that government regulations violate their freedom of speech.

The Reason Why

Why did President Clinton and Dr. Kessler target the marketing and sales of cigarettes, snuff, and chewing tobacco? Because countless studies show that children and teens are bombarded with messages and images from the tobacco industry every day of their lives. Unlike adults, children and teens

(continued on page 88)

THE STING

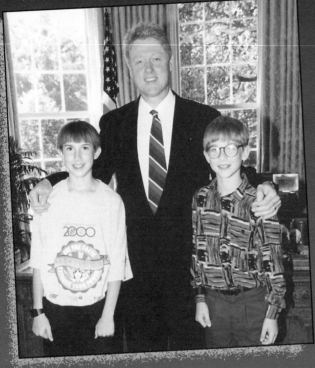

The Lesko brothers with President Clinton

In 1991, nine-year-old Morgan Lesko and his six-year-old brother, Max, staged a sting, proving that underage kids can buy cigarettes from vending machines. Here's what Morgan Lesko had to say to the Montgomery County, Maryland, council in July of 1991: "Last Friday we went to Big Boys for dinner. There we saw a vending machine. I wasn't sure what to do. So I thought about kids who really want to smoke and how they would buy cigarettes. When I finally got all the quarters in, Max pulled the handle. At least ten people were around and didn't say anything. . . ."

"That night we went to the Bowling Alley and there was another vending machine. It was wide open. I was very scared but Max wasn't. He put the quarters in but they got jammed. Then we went up to this kid Jeff who is a ninth grader at Walter Johnson High School. . . . We told him what we were doing about getting rid of vending machines. He thought it was a great idea. Then we asked him if he would help us by buying cigarettes. He just went right up to the machine with his back to about twenty people but no one cared. That night Max and I learned how to get the cigarettes easily.

The next day we went shopping at Giant. This time the machine was right next to the candy and toy vending machines. Max and I knew exactly what to do. We put the dollar bills in and pushed the buttons and got the cigarettes. And guess what, the store manager was near us and he didn't say a word."

"I think we proved that any kid can go up to a vending machine and buy cigarettes."

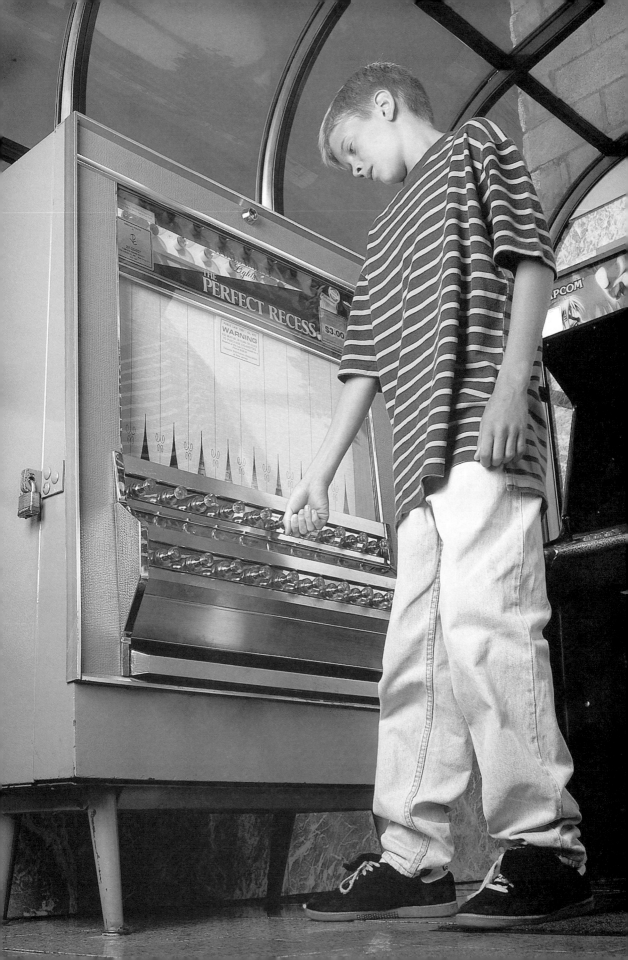

are far more likely to respond to the ads that link smoking with happiness, good looks, success, and popularity—all qualities desired by young people. Many experts have studied the links between advertising and youth and have found them to be very strong. The author of one study interviewed 3,536 young people between the ages of 12 and 17 who had never smoked. He found that when children see ads and handle cigarette packs, their resistance to smoking weakens. Later on, they will be more willing to accept a cigarette from a peer when it's offered.

In addition to having a low resistance to tobacco advertising, young people found they could easily buy smokes. By 1996, although every state had outlawed the sale of tobacco to anyone under 18, study after study showed that these laws did not put a dent in teen smoking. Teens still found it easy to buy cigarettes despite signs and stickers (part of a campaign launched by the tobacco industry) on cash registers, saying, "It's the Law: You must be 18 to buy tobacco products." Restricting sales in stores was not enough. Even though states banned the sale of tobacco to anyone under 18, young people could still often buy cigarettes from vending machines. Nobody checked. A 14-year-old girl proved the point in March 1996—right under the government's nose. The Virginia girl, lobbying in support of the FDA's proposed restrictions on tobacco advertising to children, showed she could buy a pack of cigarettes from a vending machine located in a government

In May 1997, the FTC said that ads featuring the Joe Camel cartoon character illegally promoted cigarettes to minors. In July 1997, the R.J. Reynolds Tobacco Company banished its cartoon character, although it will still appear in advertising overseas.

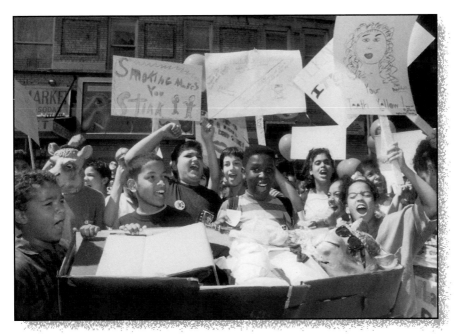

Kids bury Joe Camel

office building. When she bought the cigarettes, she was wearing a T-shirt that said "I am 14 years old."

On February 28, 1997 the FDA crackdown on tobacco sales to minors began. Federal law prohibited retailers from selling cigarettes, cigarette tobacco, or smokeless tobacco to anyone under the age of 18. Under the law retailers requested a photo ID of anyone under the age of 27. In March 2000, after the U.S. Supreme Court ruled the FDA lacked authority to regulate tobacco, photo IDs were no longer required.

Selling to the Young

About 86 percent of teen smokers buy either Marlboros, Newports, or Camels, the three most heavily advertised cigarette brands. Do they love the cigarettes or are they conned by the messages in

The original publication in 1995 of the FDA tobacco regulations triggered more mail from children than any other such publication of proposed regulations in FDA history.

When seven-year-old Sammy Blum and nine-year-old David Blum of Houston, Texas, saw that Blaze, Gambit, Kingpin, Nick Fury, and Red Skill (comic-book characters on Marvel Comics trading cards) were smoking, they got upset. Sammy wrote a letter to *The New England Journal of Medicine.* He asked: "Why do they [Marvel] make cards for kids that show people smoking?"

The journal thought Sammy had asked such an important question that it published his letter. Marvel Entertainment Group heard about the letter and thought Sammy had a good point. "There will no longer be any smoking materials depicted on the trading cards," said a Marvel Comics spokesperson. Not bad work for one seven-year-old boy.

Marvel Comics have since taken a strong antismoking stand—developing a special comic for the American Cancer Society that delivers antismoking messages.

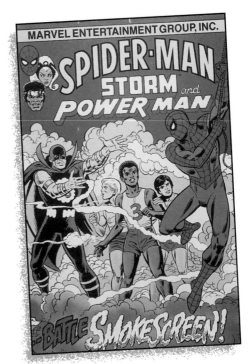

Marvel comic book for the American Cancer Society

the ads? In 1988, R. J. Reynolds launched a cartoon-like camel who quickly became as familiar to youngsters as Mickey Mouse. Joe Camel even caught the attention of some three-year-olds who were able to correctly match the cartoon camel with a picture of a cigarette. After Joe Camel was introduced, the proportion of smokers under 18 who chose Camels rose from less than 1 percent to over 30 percent!

Cartoon characters are not the only advertising gimmick to catch kids' eyes. Children and teens are strongly attracted to point-of-purchase (P-O-P) ads and displays. P-O-P advertising is done right in the drugstores, supermarkets, gas stations, or wherever cigarettes are sold. This kind of advertising includes neon signs, banners, clocks, awnings, floor and counter mats, dividers used to separate grocery orders, signs attached to display racks, signs hung from ceilings, in-store decals, ads on doors, windows, shopping carts and baskets, and checkout counters. Just take a look around when you go to the supermarket and you'll see an amazing amount of P-O-P advertising.

The Promo

Another powerful marketing gimmick that works well on young people is the promotion, or promo. In the 1990s, tobacco companies shifted some of their advertising budgets from magazines, newspapers, and billboards into promotions such as free cigarette samples or smokeless tobacco products.

Promos can also be gifts such as T-shirts, coffee mugs, lighters, ashtrays, or key chains that come wrapped with the purchase of tobacco products. They might include the appearance of a tobacco product name on TV, such as that of the Marlboro Grand Prix, and the sponsorship of community and cultural events. Promotions can also be "2 for the price of 1" specials, or coupons for free packs with the next purchase, or one or two dollars off a purchase price.

Another type of promotion has involved offering catalog merchandise in exchange for coupons from cigarette packs. More and more companies have adopted this form of advertising

In June of 1994, fifteen Horace Mann middle school students wrote a letter to the president of Philip Morris's United States operations. They protested two billboards with tobacco ads near their school, located in the Mission district of San Francisco. One billboard had a Marlboro ad; the other was a Spanish-language ad for SKOAL chewing tobacco. One sign was 140 feet from Horace Mann; the other, 505 feet away. (Philip Morris policy prevents advertising within 500 feet of a school.) The signs were removed. The campaign was coordinated by the National Latina Health Organization.

because it does not require that merchandise carry the Surgeon General's health warning. For example, Camel cigarettes offered "Camel Cash" coupons resembling one-dollar bills. These "Camel C-Notes" pictured Joe Camel in sunglasses, with a cigarette in his mouth, dressed up as George Washington. The only way you could get "the smooth stuff" pictured in Camel Cash catalogs was to collect and mail in coupons packed in Camel cigarette packs. In 1996, "Camel's Rockin' Road" CDs and cassettes cost 70 Camel C-Notes.

In 1993 and 1994, Marlboro offered logo-bearing merchandise through its "Adventure Team" promotion. Philip Morris reported that 4 million people took part, sending in coupons (called "miles") for 14 million promotional items such as team caps, sweatshirts, towels, Swiss Army knives, and rain gear. In 1996 the same company launched the "Marlboro Unlimited" campaign in which a specially built train equipped with movies, a dance club, and hot tubs was to travel through the West with 100 winners of a sweepstakes contest who testify they are smokers over 21 years of age. Needless to say, many of the catalog items made their way into the hands of young people under the age of 21. They became "walking billboards" for tobacco products.

Targeting Women and Minorities

Who are the smokers of today? Studies estimate that young women under the age of 23 are the fastest growing segment of smokers in the nation.

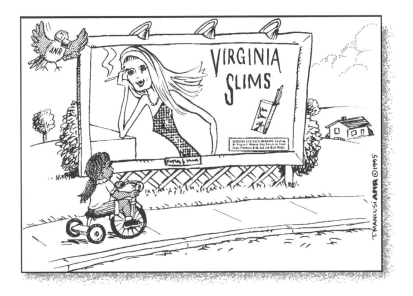

After 1967, smoking rates among girls under 17 rose sharply. That was the time when women's cigarette brands were introduced and marketed. Ads pictured thin, stylish women and used words such as slim and ultraslim to suggest that cigarettes controlled weight. When interviewed, many girls reported that they smoke to help manage their weight.

One of the biggest markets for the tobacco companies are ethnic minorities. African Americans have been a special target. In 1990, R. J. Reynolds tried to introduce a new brand of cigarettes called Uptown to the African American community in Philadelphia. African American leaders such as the Reverend Jesse Brown and Charyn Sutton formed a coalition to banish Uptown from stores in Philadelphia. They succeeded and made history. For the first time in the war on tobacco, a community was able to force a tobacco company to take a cigarette out of production. A similar story took

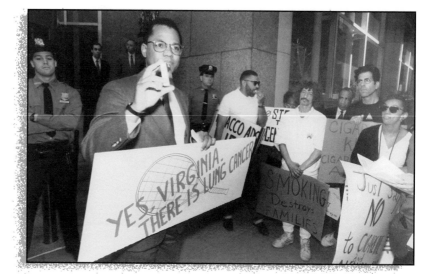

*Protesters alongside Rev. Calvin Butts,
pastor of the Abyssinian Baptist Church*

place in Boston in 1995. A brand of cigarettes called X, targeted at African Americans, was introduced in the Boston area (and in at least 19 other states). The black box, with a large white X surrounded by a red square, with "MENTHOL" spelled out in green letters, outraged many in Boston's African American community. Along with other concerned citizens throughout the nation, they demanded that production and distribution of X be stopped. Within a month, X cigarettes were removed from store shelves.

The tobacco companies run print ads in African American publications such as *Jet, Essence,* and *Ebony* as a way of capturing the African American market. Billboards advertising tobacco products are placed in predominantly African American communities four to five times more often than in white communities. In addition, tobacco companies give generously to

African American organizations, housing programs, and cultural groups. These include the Alvin Ailey Dance Theater Foundation, the Thurgood Marshall Scholarship Fund, and the National Association for the Advancement of Colored People (NAACP). In 1985, William H. Lee, publisher of the *Observer* newspapers in California, said: "Many of our black colleges would not have students receiving scholarships were it not for Philip Morris."

Tobacco companies began marketing their brands to Latino communities in the 1980s. Tobacco monies support numerous Latino publications, and many magazine and billboard ads are written in Spanish. In the Latino neighborhoods of Chicago, billboards for Newport show couples biking through scenic parks and rural countrysides beside slogans such as *Lleno de gusto* (filled with joy). Philip Morris has made contributions to organizations such as the Ballet Hispanico of New York, National Hispanic University, and National Council of La Raza. Despite their need for financial support, however, some Latino groups have turned down tobacco money. In 1991, the Mission Economic and Cultural Association (MECA), organizer of San Francisco's annual Cinco de Mayo celebration, announced it would no longer accept tobacco or alcohol sponsorship. MECA decided health costs to Latinos from tobacco and alcohol abuse were too great to accept the money that tobacco and alcohol companies made available to community events.

The enormous profits from tobacco sales allow the tobacco companies to give generously to

During the fall of 1995, Joseph Chu, Mark Cheng, and Daniel Duong (all 14 years old) conducted a sting in San Francisco's Chinatown. They went to 20 Chinatown shops and were able to buy cigarettes 52 percent of the time. The youth, members of Chinese Power Against Tobacco/Chinese Progressive Association, talked about their experiences before a meeting of the San Francisco Board of Supervisors.

a variety of Native American and other organizations. Philip Morris has contributed to the First Nations Development Institute and the American Indian College Fund. Tobacco companies fund civil liberties causes; health, religious and charitable groups; community service; and nonprofit cultural organizations. For example, Philip Morris donated $50,000 for a meeting room in a children's science museum in Charlotte, North Carolina. It's called the Philip Morris room, and smoking is permitted in it. The tobacco industry makes substantial contributions to AIDS service organizations and other groups desperate for funding. Once an organization receives such valuable funding, it does not want to lose it. Rarely do groups that receive tobacco monies criticize the industry that supports them.

The Clout of Tobacco

The tobacco industry, like many other groups, tries to influence political leaders, from both major parties. Tobacco companies are among the top campaign contributors at national and state levels. Since 1985, the industry has contributed millions of dollars to congressional campaigns, presidential campaigns, political action committees, and political party committees. The tobacco industry has been the single biggest supporter of the Republican National Committee. Many of the recipients of tobacco money have been politicians from states where tobacco is grown, foundations associated with elected officials, and the favorite charities of politicians. In 1993, a research group concluded that

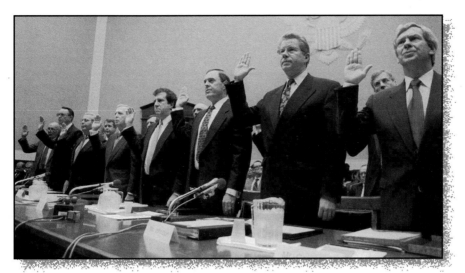

In 1994, chairmen of leading tobacco companies testified before Congress that nicotine is not addictive, and that no one has proven that tobacco products cause cancer.

tobacco contributions had a "direct" relationship to lawmakers' positions on tobacco control issues.

Despite all the advertising, promotions, sponsorships, and contributions to dozens of organizations, the tobacco industry faces an increasingly hostile reaction to smoking. Smoking restrictions have increased to include airplanes, trains, and buses. Smoking is increasingly restricted in hospitals, workplaces, restaurants, malls, college dorms, and other places. Tobacco makers are under intense legal attacks, too. The U.S. Justice Department is conducting at least five investigations of the tobacco industry. One inquiry has to do with the 1994 testimony of tobacco executives who swore that they did not believe nicotine was addictive. Prosecutors are trying to determine whether the tobacco officials lied or tried to obstruct the congressional inquiry. By September 1996, tobacco

THE DANGERS OF CHEW

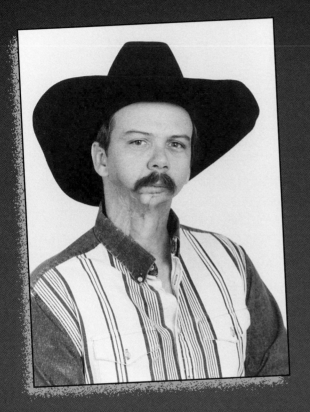

Rick Bender, of Roundup, Montana, a longtime sandlot ballplayer, flies all over the nation to show his face—or what is left of it. Why? Because he wants to warn young people about the dangers of spit (chewing) tobacco. He began dipping Copenhagen Snuff in high school and graduated to one can a day. Chewing tobacco and playing baseball seemed to go hand in hand. But in 1988, at 26, he was diagnosed with cancer. Bender had to undergo long operations to remove lymph nodes, portions of his neck and tongue, and a piece of his jaw. He only has two teeth left in the lower part of his mouth. He also lost some use of his right arm from nerve damage and can't throw a baseball or swing a bat.

This is Rick Bender's message: "I'm 33 years old now, but at the age of 26 I was diagnosed with cancer. Because of the cancer and infections and treatment, I lost one half of my jaw and one third of my tongue. Why did this happen to me? Because when I was young, I got into the habit of chewing tobacco.

If you chew or know someone who does, and any of you get a sore in your mouth that doesn't go away in ten days, get it checked out. Early detection is the best way of avoiding a catastrophe like mine.

If I can keep even one student from each school from st___ this terrible habit and ___ugh what I have, it will __t."

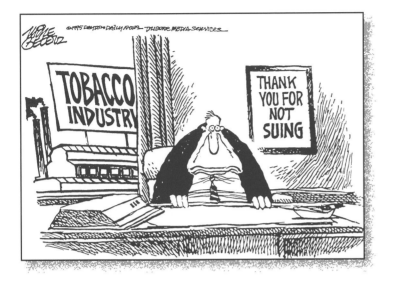

companies faced lawsuits in at least 23 states. The attorneys general of those states argued that the tobacco companies should bear the medical costs for their poorest patients with smoking-related diseases. In 1997, the number of states suing the tobacco industry rose, to 40.

Tobacco companies are not only dealing with lawsuits. They are also dealing with former employees who have "blown the whistle" on secret tobacco-company documents that imply tobacco companies knew their products were addictive and manipulated nicotine levels. Former researchers and scientists for the tobacco companies have made statements on national television and to lawyers about the inner workings of Philip Morris and of Brown & Williamson. Many of the documents and statements from former tobacco employees could be used as evidence in the lawsuits.

In 1997, the nation's smallest major cigarette

maker, the Liggett Group, Inc., settled with 22 states and hundreds of smokers. It acknowledged smoking causes cancer and other diseases and agreed to stamp "Warning: Smoking is Addictive" on Chesterfield, Eve, and its other brands.

In November 1998 the attorney generals of 46 states and the five largest cigarette companies reached an historic settlement over state health costs for treating sick smokers. The tobacco companies agreed to pay $206 billion over 25 years to 46 states and five U.S. territories. The money can be spent on anything state legislatures decide. (Mississippi, Florida, Texas, and Minnesota separately settled their claims with major cigarette producers). The agreement banned billboard and transit ads after April 1999 and banned merchandise with cigarette brand logos. The tobacco companies agreed to pay for tobacco-cessation programs and to create the American Legacy Foundation that researches ways to reduce youth smoking.

The war on tobacco companies has heated up. In July 2000 a Florida jury ordered the tobacco-industry to pay a record award of $145 billion to sick Florida smokers. The tobacco companies pledged to fight the verdict. They have the resources and the clout. You have the information to make your own decision.

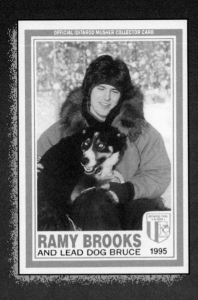

In keeping with the purpose of the first Iditarod (a trail sled-dog race), which brought life-saving diphtheria serum to Nome, Alaska, the race in recent years has been used to raise public awareness about modern health plagues including alcohol and AIDS. In 1995, a new cause was added. Musher Ramy Brooks carried a message aimed at reducing the number-one cause of death in rural Alaska—tobacco use.

Brooks, a 26-year-old musher of Athabaskan and Eskimo ancestry from Fairbanks, Alaska, won Rookie of the Year honors in 1994 for his seventeenth place finish. He placed 8th in the race in 1997.

When the Alaska Native Health Board sent a notice out to all the 1995 Iditarod mushers, looking for someone to carry a "tobacco-free" message, Brooks, who has raced dogs since the age of four, was the first to respond.

Brooks passed out a specially designed "musher collector card" to his fans during the 1995 Iditarod. The card features a photograph of Brooks and his lead dog Bruce on the front, and the Trampling Tobacco logo on the back. The logo shows a husky in harness trampling cigarettes and chewing tobacco into the snow. Brooks displayed the same logo in full color on his clothing and sled bag. Buttons that read "Trampling Tobacco with Ramy Brooks" were sent to schools along the Iditarod route. Brooks also starred in a television public-service announcement (PSA) with the message "It's great to be tobacco-free!" The project appealed to Brooks because as he says "the decisions you make when you're young and the identity you develop set the stage for everything that comes later. Being tobacco-free needs to be part of that identity."

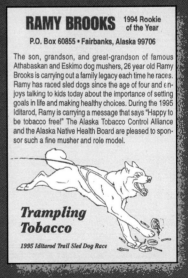

RAMY BROOKS 1994 Rookie of the Year

P.O. Box 60855 • Fairbanks, Alaska 99706

The son, grandson, and great-grandson of famous Athabaskan and Eskimo dog mushers, 26 year old Ramy Brooks is carrying out a family legacy each time he races. Ramy has raced sled dogs since the age of four and enjoys talking to kids today about the importance of setting goals in life and making healthy choices. During the 1995 Iditarod, Ramy is carrying a message that says "Happy to be tobacco free!" The Alaska Tobacco Control Alliance and the Alaska Native Health Board are pleased to sponsor such a fine musher and role model.

Trampling Tobacco

1995 Iditarod Trail Sled Dog Race

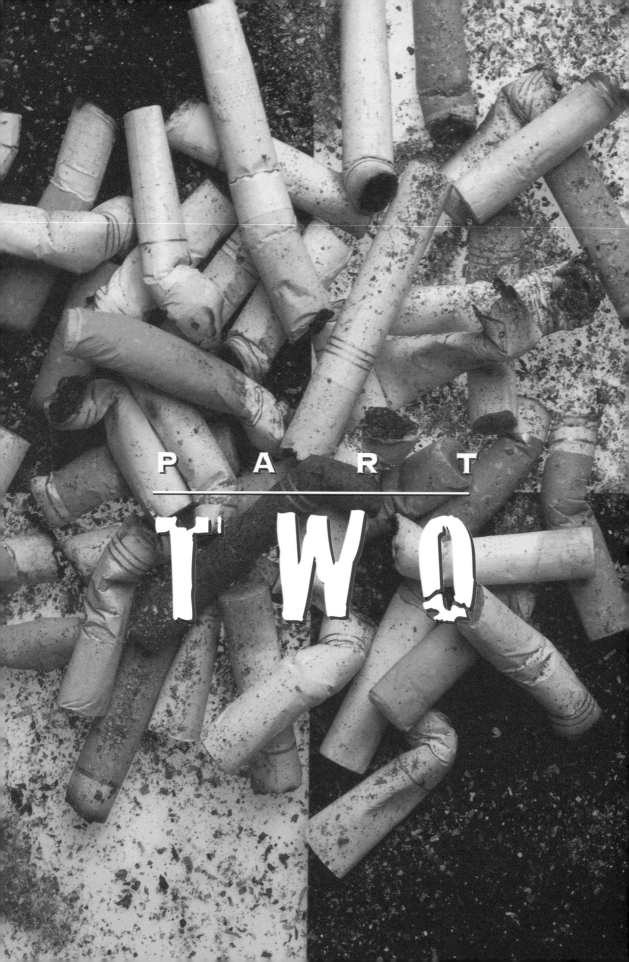

PART

TWO

Kids
Kick
Butts

Knowing the history of tobacco and cigarette smoking is one way to help yourself stay smoke-free. Another way is to read about young people all over the country who run smoke-free activities. Maybe some of these programs will tempt you to try them in your own community.

Smoke-Filled Bathrooms

- You need a gas mask to get into some of the smoke-filled bathrooms in schools throughout the nation. At Magruder High School in Rockville, Maryland, there was so much smoking going on that school officials locked the bathroom doors.

  For some students, a puffless bathroom is a matter of life and death. In 1995, the parents of Heather Morris, a Tinely Park High School junior in Chicago, Illinois, sued the school because officials there failed to stop her classmates from smoking in the girls' bathrooms. Smoking can kill Heather, who has severe asthma. The suit is among the first to test an Illinois law that prohibits smoking on school property. Stay tuned.

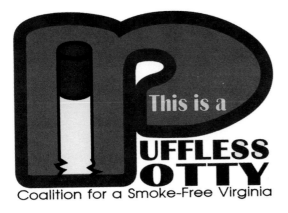

This is a **PUFFLESS POTTY**

Coalition for a Smoke-Free Virginia

- In Virginia, students helped design "Puffless Potty" stickers to remind fellow students that bathrooms are for something other than breathing cigarette smoke.

Smoke-Free Schools

- In San Jose, California, teens circulated a petition to make their schools smoke-free. They gathered over 800 signatures. After presenting their petition to the school board, the superintendent of schools was directed to develop a policy to ban tobacco use on ten high school campuses.

- April Swartz, a student at Sandwich Junior/Senior High School in Sandwich, Massachusetts, challenged state lawmakers with this argument: "If someone came to you asking to stop teen suicide, everyone would be in favor of that idea. Our bill is the first step in slowing down a form of teen suicide."

   April was one of nearly 30 students from her high school who lobbied Massachusetts lawmakers to pass a law making public school grounds in the state tobacco-free. It took two years to get the law passed, but the teens won. With the help of William Sangster, a health education teacher, they organized Sandwich Students Against Smoking. In the process, they learned how to write letters to lawmakers, give interviews to reporters, do face-to-face lobbying with legislators, and offer informed testimony at the state capitol. According to Mr. Sangster, the law enacted in 1987 "was the only piece of legislation ever passed in the history of the Massachusetts legislature sponsored directly by kids."

The Young Ad-Team

- Six-year-old Jackie Love is not your usual advertising copywriter. In 1994, Jackie's slogan, "Save Someone Special: Stop Smoking!" beat out those of over 900 Billerica, Massachusetts, students. The youngsters were taking part in a contest for elementary students to create a short, catchy slogan for an antitobacco campaign. Jackie's advertising agency, the Billerica Ad Lab, is located in the Billerica school district. It provides students and teachers with the chance to plan, design, create, and release public-service announcements (PSAs). It produced 20,000 stickers and T-shirts bearing Jackie's slogan and urged students to create PSAs using Jackie's theme. Nearly 2,000 students submitted editorials, cartoons, rap songs, bumper stickers, videos, signs, and drawings. The PSAs were videotaped and shown on the local access television station, and the editorials appeared on a special page in the school newspaper. The award-winning poster by 12-year old Jonathan

Renoni ended up on a town billboard! Not bad work for what the Boston media called "the youngest advertising team in the business."

Seventeen-Year-Old Sues

- In 1987, seventeen-year-old Theresa Kyte and her father sued Philip Morris and Store 24 of Waltham, Massachusetts. The reason? Theresa was ill and nicotine-dependent. She blamed the cigarette maker and the store for conspiring to sell cigarettes to minors like herself. Theresa had been buying her cigarettes, made by Philip Morris, from Store 24 since she was 14, despite a state law prohibiting cigarette sales to people under 18. Theresa's lawsuit also said that Philip Morris had conspired to increase its profits and "hook" a new generation of smokers. Philip Morris tried to get the case dismissed, but failed. In 1991 the Massachusetts Supreme Judicial Court decided the cigarette maker has no control over the stores that sell its products. However, a judge did rule that retailers are liable for any nicotine addiction that customers suffer from cigarettes. As part of the settlement, Store 24 promised to closely monitor its sales to prevent kids under 18 from buying cigarettes.

The War Against Vending Machines

- High school students in Salem, Massachusetts, were concerned about the ease with which kids were buying cigarettes from vending machines. They proposed a law to ban cigarette vending machines in Salem. The idea for the ban started in a health class, and eventually 300 students joined the campaign. The teens collected 1,400 signatures and filed a proposal for a city ordinance with the city clerk. The city council agreed to discuss the proposal, and the ordinance passed in 1994. "I didn't think we could influence city government as much as we did," said one Salem student, "and that made me think we have more power over what happens in our city, especially to people our own age."

- In northern California, teens in Marin and Santa Clara counties took part in surveys to document illegal sales of tobacco products to minors. They shared the results with city councils, which then banned cigarette vending machines in their communities.

Smoke-Free Malls

- In Chicopee, Massachusetts, members of the Student Tobacco Opposition Program (STOP) thought their local mall had some pretty cool shops, but the secondhand smoke there was definitely uncool. They talked to the head of the mall about it and challenged the local board of health to take action. The youngsters got a referendum on the city ballot. Chicopee voters approved the move to make the mall smoke-free. STOP's work on behalf of a smoke-free environment continued. It then persuaded all restaurants in Chicopee to become smoke-free, too.

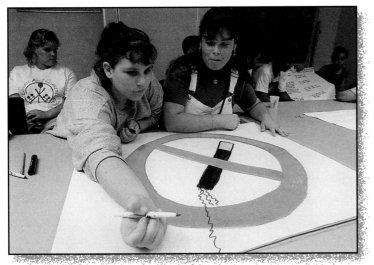

Teens' antismoking campaign, Chicopee, Massachusetts

The activities of STOP have brought the group a lot of attention. In 1995, STOP presented a workshop at the annual Stop Teenage Addiction to Tobacco (STAT) Conference and was honored for its leadership and antitobacco involvement. It has also consulted with a newly formed Australian antitobacco youth group called QUIT.

Kids Sting Tobacco Sellers

• As part of an after-school project on teen smoking, a group of sixth, seventh, and eighth graders from Elm Place School in Highland Park, Illinois, decided to "sting" local merchants who sold cigarettes to them. After school, Suzanne Greenwald, an Elm Place teacher and project director, drove her students to Highland Park businesses that sold cigarettes. Students took turns going into these stores to buy cigarettes. Greenwald videotaped each student coming out of a store, often with cigarettes in hand. In some instances, the student would tell the store clerk, "I do not have identification," and still get a pack. Out of 17 attempts by the students to buy cigarettes from a sales clerk or a vending machine, 12 were successful. But the kids didn't want to name the business owners who had sold them cigarettes illegally. They wanted the community to know there was a problem that needed fixing. The problem was fixed. The city council passed a law that prohibits the sale of tobacco to minors as well as its possession by minors. The law also calls for periodic and unannounced visits to stores by underage high school volunteers working with the police department. Kids found in possession of tobacco would be given a ticket similar to a parking ticket.

- In August 1996, eighth grader Anna Santiago, one of the students involved in Suzanne Greenwald's project, got a call from the White House. Before she knew it, Anna was in Washington, D.C., seated next to President Clinton in a White House Rose Garden ceremony. The President was there to announce restrictions on tobacco advertising and sales to youngsters. To top her day, Anna received the "Advocate of the Year" award from the Campaign for Tobacco-Free Kids for her work in Highland Park.

Teen Media

- "By Children for Everybody" is the motto of Children's Express (CE), a monthly youth news service and leadership organization devoted to

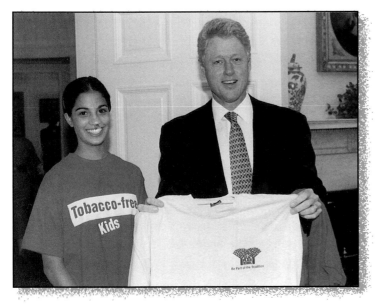

Anna Santiago with President Clinton

giving children a voice in the world. Through tape-recorded interviews, commentaries, and round-table discussions, young reporters between the ages of 8 and 13 and young editors 14 through 18 report on issues important to youth and adults alike. Their news service provides copy to newspapers around the world and works on various book projects. Children's Express, located in Washington, D.C., has been in business for over 20 years.

In January 1995, Teen Express, a division of Children's Express, interviewed David Kessler, the FDA commissioner.

TE: What do you want to do to stop kids from smoking?

DK: We need to reduce the easy access to cigarettes. Ask a teenager who smokes whether it's easy to buy cigarettes and he or she'll say "yes." What a lot of teenagers say to me is, "If this was so bad for you, you wouldn't have it right out there so that I could buy it that easily."

TE: Does the FDA really have the right to restrict or regulate this if someone's in the privacy of their own home?

DK: There are laws that limit advertising of drugs. That's what we do at the Food and Drug Administration. There are laws that don't allow just anyone to advertise or to say anything they want about any drug. Our job is to look at the question of nicotine and whether that's a drug. How do you restrict access to that product so people don't become addicted? That's our job.

TE: What is your ultimate goal?

DK: The goal is to reduce the number of children who become addicted.

- "Youth Radio" is a multicultural broadcast journalism training program for teens in Berkeley, California, founded in 1992. Youth Radio offers teens a place in the media to voice their own ideas, passions, and concerns. Jacinda Abcarian, a reporter with Youth Radio, talked to teens who are as doubtful about the government's efforts to keep them from smoking as they are about the sales pitches from the tobacco industry. Here's a short excerpt from "Teens and Cigarettes," in which Jacinda Abcarian interviews a teen who began smoking at an early age. It originally aired on National Public Radio's *All Things Considered* (a news show) on December 27, 1995.

  JA: Throughout high school, I watched as many of my friends tried to balance going to class and "fiending" for the next hit. "Fiending" is just an expression my friends and I use to describe how crazed smokers get when they are looking for a cigarette. The teens I know don't see that much difference between cigarettes and other drugs. . . .

Student: I was about 11 or 12, in junior high, and basically I hung out with a lot of older people. That's what they did, so that's what I started doin'—on and off.

JA: You said that everyone had cigarettes. So where did you go about getting your cigarettes?

Student: The stores. I mean, they did have vending machines, but they're expensive. So it's not like they card you or anything. So we just used to go in the store and buy the cigarettes and, if not, you see a bum hanging outside. You give a quarter and they'll go buy 'em for you. It's not hard.

Puff, the Magic Wagon

Gretchen Campbell is a Paducah, Kentucky, teenager who rides a most unusual school bus. Art students at Heath High School in Paducah transformed an ordinary school bus into "Puff, the Magic Wagon," a mobile classroom filled with teaching displays such as "Smokey Sue," "Mr. Dip Lip™," and "Mr. Gross Mouth.™" On board are Gretchen and other teen teachers who travel from elementary school to elementary school with a smoke-free message. Here's how Gretchen describes the project.

> In the state of Kentucky, which is the tobacco capital of the world, there is my small school of about 600 students in my small town, called Paducah. Ironically, my school, which sits right next to a tobacco barn, is involved in trying to prevent the smoking and chewing of tobacco. We are trying to get to the children early on, and try to put into their innocent minds the idea that smoking and chewing are not cool and should not be tried. . . . Being in a state where the pressures of smoking are

greater than usual, it isn't easy to teach little kids when everyone in their environment smokes.

Each one of the high school students involved in Tobacco Education is assigned and responsible for knowing about a display and explaining the importance of it to the children. "Smokey Sue" is used to show students the effects of the cigarette and the amount of tar that collects in your lungs. "Mr. Dip Lip™" and "Mr. Gross Mouth™" both explain the harmful and disgusting results of chewing tobacco and smoking. "The Smoker's Roulette" is another display in which the object of the game is not to play. If you play—you smoke or chew—you lose. If you don't play— don't smoke or chew—you win. As children play the game, they get information on what happens to your body from smoking or chewing.

Teens as Teachers

- Teenagers are effective teachers of the smoke-free message. And they are not afraid of looking silly while telling others about the dangers of smoking. "Don't clown around with tobacco" is the message student clowns from Brooke High School in West Virginia give to younger children. The photo of the clowns appeared in the school newspaper as well as in high school football programs.

- In Massachusetts, in the Mission Hill district of Boston, *Jovenes Latinos en Acion Contra el Tabaco* ("Youth in Action Against Tobacco") presented some eye-opening information to convenience store operators and other merchants in Boston. The teens showed store owners the results of a community survey along with a map showing the presence of billboards and other tobacco ads. They explained how tobacco ads and the sale of cigarettes contribute to youth smoking. Merchants responded favorably because the students presented their information in a spirit of collaboration.

The group also works directly with teens and children, providing tobacco education to local schools and presenting workshops in Casa Isla, a residential home for young men. The teen leaders have found that when they show the true cost of tobacco gear, comparing the money spent on packs of cigarettes to the same money the kids would pay in a store for merchandise, the young people really pay attention.

- Each year, the "Thunder on the Ohio" boat race is held in Indiana. Recently, Indiana teens voiced their opposition to Camels' sponsorship of the race. To send a positive message, the teens sponsored a tobacco-prevention float in a parade held nearby. The youngsters gave away T-shirts and drink-holders—the same kind of promos tobacco companies offer, except the kids' giveaways had a smoke-free message.

Stars Don't Make the Grade

- In Humble, Texas, the students at Pine Forest Elementary School give grades to movie stars based on whether they are good role models for children. The students fill out real report cards to send to movie stars who smoke in films. Among the stars who got all "Fs" are Jim Carey, Brad Renfro, Brittany Murphy, and Melanie Griffith. The idea started with Lucy Richardson, the school nurse. Her efforts have won her an award from the Texas state health commissioner, who wants to develop Lucy's report cards and other activities into an antismoking pilot project to be used statewide.

Let's Talk About Smoke, Baby

(Sung)
Let's talk about
smoke, baby.
Let's talk about
the lungs in me.
Let's talk about
all the bad things
that could happen
if you're not smoke free.
Let's talk about smoke.
Let's talk about smoke.

(Spoken)
Smoking causes you
to make mistakes.
Smoking ruins your lungs.
Smoking brings you
closer to death.
Smoking is unpopular.
Smoking ruins your life.
Pam, Stephanie, Kim,
Tameka, Tara.
We all choose to be
smoke free
and we hope you do, too.

- In many states, kids are performing and broadcasting their smoke-free tunes. In Richmond, Virginia, a team of five students from Brookland Middle School won a radio public-service announcement contest. Sixth-grade students from schools across the state submitted cassettes of 30-second spots carrying smoke-free messages. The words from the winning entry are shown at left.

- In New Jersey, Mike Dellapia, who was a junior at South Plainfield High School, quit smoking and joined a "Teens as Teachers" project. Mike quit because smoking hurt his drum-playing in a heavy metal band. Mike's teaching team drew on his music background to create a rap they performed for younger kids. (shown on the next page)

PSA (Public-Service Announcement)

- In Alaska, Elmer J. "E. J." Howarth, a sixth grader from the Inupiat village of Noatak, won a statewide radio PSA contest. The "Trampling Tobacco" project sponsored the contest, which asked writers to combine the theme of the Iditarod Trail Sled Dog Race with a tobacco prevention theme. E.J., whose family raises sled dogs, was selected the grand prize winner after beating out over 130 entrants. His winning PSA was aired on the radio during the Iditarod to over 300 small communities around the state, including E.J.'s own village. E.J. won a trip to Anchorage to see the start of the race, meet Ramy Brooks, and record his PSA at Alaska Public Radio Network Studios. Here's Elmer J. Howarth's PSA.

> Be a winner. You can be a champion just like the famous Iditarod dogs. Don't smoke cigarettes. Mush your way to healthy lungs. The dogs need healthy lungs to run in the Iditarod. Tobacco can hurt our bodies. Tobacco can give us cancer and get our lungs black. Ramy Brooks in the Iditarod does not smoke or chew because he has to be healthy. People think chewing tobacco and smoking tobacco is cool. It is sad. The only way Iditarod dogs would stop running is when they get old. When smokers stop doing something, it's probably because they get sick or die from cancer.

Posters, Posters Everywhere

- Children and teens are creating posters advising teens to be smoke-free that are showing up in subway stations, on community billboards, on book jackets, in books about tobacco issues, and in school hallways. Around the nation, students carry antismoking posters in antismoking protests.

- In Brooklyn, New York, five-year-old Erin Fels created a poster that ended up as the official logo of the SmokeLess State program. Erin's poster and message—"Smoking is Bad, It is Garbage"—appears

"Don't Smoke Rap"

My name is Leroy
and I don't smoke
and I never will
'Cause I know smoke
is dangerous
and it could kill.

Her name is Laurie
and she's a dancer,
And she don't smoke
'cause she don't want cancer.

My name is Steve.
I know smoking ain't cool
I tried it once and
I felt like a fool.

My name is Mike,
I used to smoke
But I quit cold turkey
because I know
it's no joke.

I'm big daddy Al
but I'm not proud
Because smoking makes
a nasty cloud.

Her name is Jenny B.
and that's no joke
She's a real athlete
cause she doesn't smoke!

117

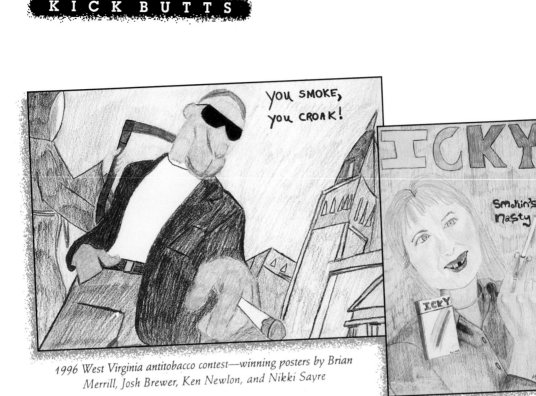

YOU SMOKE, YOU CROAK!

ICKY

Smokin's nasty

ICKY

1996 West Virginia antitobacco contest—winning posters by Brian Merrill, Josh Brewer, Ken Newlon, and Nikki Sayre

on the SmokeLess State T-shirt. Kids from nineteen states that took part in this national tobacco control and prevention program wear their shirts at smoke-free events.

- In Albuquerque, New Mexico, students took part in a tobacco-prevention poster contest. They asked merchants near their school to display the winning posters. Many store owners took part and helped deliver a strong message to all.

Murals, Too

- Children and teens are battling tobacco companies on a big scale. They are working with professional artists to warn their communities about the dangers of smoking.

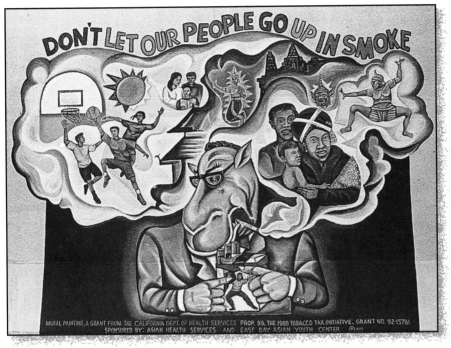

Mural of Joe Camel at Roosevelt Jr. High School, East Oakland, CA

• In East Oakland, California, a mural on a wall near Roosevelt Junior High School warns the community "Don't Let Our People Go Up in Smoke." It is the first Asian antitobacco mural in the predominately Asian East Bay area. For six weeks, youth employed by the East Bay Asian Youth Center planned and painted the mural with Filipino American muralist Orlando Castillo. The mural shows a big-nosed camel puffing a cigarette. Smoke encircles his head, and in this smoke are pictures of Asian youths playing basketball, a couple watching as their son reads, temples, and a mask. According to Yin Yan Leung, the coordinator of the tobacco program of Asian Health Services, (a sponsor of the mural project), there is a very high rate of smoking among

119

Asians. According to the Alameda County Tobacco Control Program, many Asian Americans are not aware of the hazards of smoking. In a survey conducted in Oakland's Chinatown section, 40 percent of Chinese men did not know that smoking caused heart disease.

In Berkeley, California, a group of nine Berkeley High School student artists painted a brilliantly colored mural on the south side of the school's B building. It took 23 days to complete. Professional muralist Corinne Guiney provided direction. The nine Berkeley student artists tried to get across the idea that teens are being manipulated. They painted a genderless figure they named "the addict" in the center of the mural. A smiling Joe Camel holds the figure in chains. A cigarette package clutching handfuls of cash tramples on a kid that it controls through his own addiction. Around the painted scenes is a border with the names of some of the 4,000 chemicals released when tobacco is smoked or chewed.

Teen Theater

- Young actors are taking the smoke-free message to audiences in live performances. In Coachella, California, Teen Teatro has entertained over 3,500 young people with its tobacco-education program. Teen actors developed scripts based on realistic experiences that young audiences can relate to.

- Thirteen high school and college students from California's San Diego County make up the

Anti-Tobacco Action Campaign team (ATAC). ATAC's young actors take antitobacco messages to elementary and middle school children. They base their skits on popular television shows such as *Batman* and *Pinky and the Brain.* ATAC helps young audiences understand that tobacco is a "Poison Pool," that secondhand smoke is a "Haze Maze," and that tobacco advertising is a deceptive "Bait Plate," not one to eat from.

Young Animators

- Did you see *The Lion King?* Do you love those reruns of *Looney Tunes?* If so, then you appreciate the animator's art. Young animators around the nation are creating smoke-free messages by using this famous art form.

- In Oakland, California, a group of young Asians and Pacific Islanders, ages 8 to 18, made their own animated antitobacco cartoons. They learned the basics at a two-day cartoon-making workshop led by AnimAction, a cartoon production company. Five 30-second cartoons made by the kids premiered at the East Bay Youth Center. The cartoons were used as TV public-service announcements and in educational presentations in the community.

- African American students from John B. Turner Middle School in Philadelphia teamed up with professional animator and filmmaker John Serpentelli to create "Smoking on the Hush, Hush Tip," a five-minute film. The youngsters learned animation techniques, script writing, and the art of collage making. The students created their own mixed-media collages, wrote the scripts, and recorded the narration for the antismoking film. A reviewer for the *Philadelphia Review* praised the student film as "a vigorous work with a powerful message and highly attractive images."

Youth Leadership Conferences

- Youngsters are getting smarter and smarter about smoking and tobacco issues. They attend the growing number of youth conferences held around the nation.

- In New Mexico, hundreds of high school students attended a peer-leadership conference on substance-abuse prevention. They attended workshops and panel discussions, created tobacco-free commercials, worked on a gigantic antitobacco collage, and performed in a talent contest. The students got to meet model and former Winston Man David B. Goerlitz, who appeared in 42 Winston cigarette ads. In 1988, Goerlitz took a historic stand against the tobacco industry. He condemned the targeting and selling of tobacco products to young people.

- Young people from the Pauma Valley Indian Reservation attended a youth leadership conference in North Escondido, California. The Escondido Community Health Center's Tobacco-Free Living Communities (TLC) trained them to serve as role models for their peers and to become decision makers in the community. The youth meet every

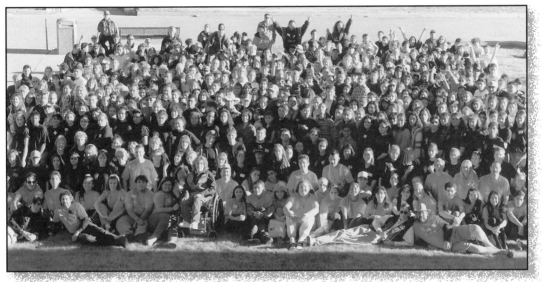

6th annual New Mexico peer-leadership conference

other week to plan and carry out their activities. TLC assists them with ideas toward creating tobacco-free environments.

Look-alikes Take a Hike

- In Elsie, Michigan, elementary school students didn't like the messages they saw in the sale of candy cigarettes that look just like real cigarette brands. Fourth graders wrote to their state senator about the fake cigarettes. They got a letter back, along with a copy of a study that links candy cigarettes with later use of real cigarettes. Students visited all the stores in the area and convinced three managers to change their store policies and stop selling the candy. The students were helped by a TV station and a newspaper, both of which featured their campaign.

123

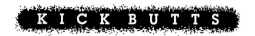

Surgeon General's Warning, Seventh-Grade Style

- In Maine, some seventh-grade students studied the Surgeon General's warnings that appear on all ads, cigarette packs, and spit tobacco. They came up with some catchy messages that wound up being published in the local newspaper.

> **SURGEON GENERAL'S WARNING: If you smoke, you'll choke, then croak, so don't be a DOPE!**

> **SURGEON GENERAL'S WARNING: Smoking will cause social problems, health complications, and death. Quit now or forever hold your breath.**

> **SURGEON GENERAL'S WARNING: Smoking doesn't just empty your life, it empties your wallet.**

Student Coalition Against Tobacco (SCAT)

- The Student Coalition Against Tobacco (SCAT) is a teen activist organization. It was formed early in 1993 by David Dubner and Scott Marcus. David and Scott started a smoke-free movement within the Wantagh School District on Long Island, New York. Students rallied to rid their school of second-hand smoke coming from the teachers' smoking lounge. The group was successful in their efforts—the entire school eventually became smoke-free.

SCAT was founded by youth, for youth, and is operated by youth. Board members range in age from 13 to 23. Here's how SCAT explains itself.

> As an organization led and directed by youth, we are in a very good position to address the needs of our constituency. SCAT members are immersed throughout the target population—SCAT serves their own. Therefore, a high degree of accessibility to our constituency exists. SCAT, along with every step of the program, will be visible, definite, and witnessed by youth since these activities will take place within their domain. The mere presence of SCAT, as the only youth-led organization dedicated to tobacco issues, will have a profound effect within the youth community.

TOBACCO
FACTS

What's in Tobacco and How
It Affects Your Health

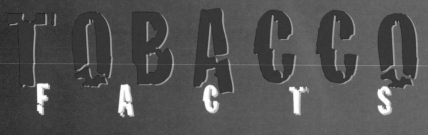

Basic Tobacco Facts

The leafy tobacco plant is a member of the vegetable family Solanaceae. The plant was named *Nicotiana tabacum* in honor of Jean Nicot, the French ambassador to Portugal in the 1580s. Nicot thought the plant had medicinal value and encouraged its cultivation.

In the United States, tobacco is grown from New Hampshire to Florida and as far west as Minnesota. As a result of differences in soil, climate, and plant varieties, each region produces a different kind and quality of leaf.

The main ingredient in cigarettes is tobacco, which comes from the leaves of various species of *Nicotiana*, a member of the nightshade family. In the United States, the tobacco plant *Nicotiana tabacum* is used primarily for the manufacture of cigarettes, cigars, pipe tobaccos, and to a lesser extent, chewing tobacco. As in most agriculture, various herbicides, pesticides, and insecticides are used to kill unwanted weeds, diseases, and insects. These chemicals find their way into tobacco products.

Green tobacco leaf is "cured" to develop the taste and aroma desired by users of the various products. In air-curing, the tobacco is sheltered in barns but cured primarily under natural weather conditions. In flue-curing, the tobacco is cured in heated air but not subjected to smoke or odors. In fire-curing, the tobacco is cured by wood fires and smoke that come in direct contact with tobacco leaves.

Flue-cured tobacco is the principal type used in North America. It forms almost the whole content of cigarettes and a large part of the ingredients of pipe tobaccos. Only shade-grown cigar-wrapper leaf is more intensely cultivated. Flue-cured tobacco is produced in the states of Florida, Georgia, Virginia, North Carolina, and South Carolina.

Dark-fired tobacco is a large, heavy kind of leaf grown in denser soil than flue-cured tobacco is. It was first grown in Virginia and Kentucky. It is also grown in Tennessee.

Burley and other air-cured tobaccos are grown in naturally fertile limestone soil. Burley, grown mainly in Kentucky, is widely used in the United States both for cigarettes and pipe mixtures.

Cigar tobaccos are grown in Connecticut. Once virtually all cigars were made from West Indian and Cuban leaves. Cigar tobacco is air-cured.

Most of the popular brand cigarettes consist of a blend of flue-cured, Burley, Maryland, and Turkish tobaccos. Some cigarettes are made wholly of flue-cured tobaccos and some of Turkish alone. The term "Turkish" is misleading. "Turkish" tobacco comes not only from Turkey but also from Greece, Bulgaria, and other Mediterranean countries and islands. It is an aromatic, light-colored, air-cured type and is sometimes called the "pepper and salt" or "seasoning" of cigarettes.

What's in Cigarette and Tobacco Smoke

Tobacco smoke contains thousands of elements. Most of these are delivered in such small amounts that they are not usually considered in discussions of the health effects of cigarette smoking. There are three elements, however, that are always discussed as health hazards of smoking cigarettes: nicotine, tar, and carbon monoxide. Tar and carbon monoxide are not even present in an unburned cigarette. They are produced when a puff is taken.

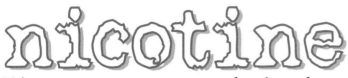

Tobacco contains nicotine, one of a class of compounds called alkaloids. The class also includes cocaine and morphine. Tobacco plants produce nicotine as a toxic chemical defense against insects.

Nicotine is a potent drug that occurs naturally in the leaves of *Nicotiana tabacum*. It is one of the most harmful poisons known. One drop of it in a concentrated state is enough to kill a dog. Eight drops of nicotine will kill a horse in four minutes. Nicotine does not kill the smoker because it is absorbed over a period of time. The body breaks its down and eliminates it in urine.

Nicotine is absorbed by the body at remarkable speed. After a smoker inhales cigarette smoke into his or her lungs, nicotine transfers directly from the tiny airholes in the lungs into the bloodstream. From there, inhaled nicotine rushes to the brain in less than 10 seconds. It reaches the big toe in 15 to 20 seconds. It is also well absorbed through the

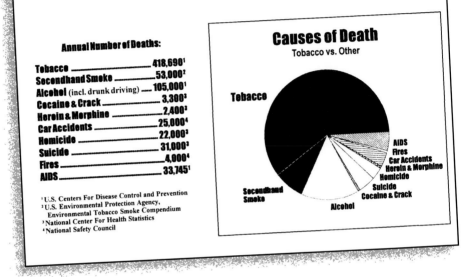

Tobacco Kills More Americans Each Year Than Alcohol, Cocaine, Crack, Heroin, Car Accidents, Homicide, Suicide, Fires, and AIDS *combined.*

Annual Number of Deaths:

Tobacco	418,690[1]
Secondhand Smoke	53,000[2]
Alcohol (incl. drunk driving)	105,000[1]
Cocaine & Crack	3,300[3]
Heroin & Morphine	2,400[3]
Car Accidents	25,000[4]
Homicide	22,000[3]
Suicide	31,000[3]
Fires	4,000[4]
AIDS	33,745[1]

[1] U.S. Centers For Disease Control and Prevention
[2] U.S. Environmental Protection Agency, Environmental Tobacco Smoke Compendium
[3] National Center For Health Statistics
[4] National Safety Council

Causes of Death
Tobacco vs. Other

very thin skin of the mouth or the nose, which is dense with capillaries. That is why chewing tobacco and inhaling snuff are such effective ways to take in nicotine.

Nicotine is an addictive drug. Some experts say it is the most addictive drug there is—more so than heroin or alcohol. It affects mood, feeling, and behavior by entering the brain and causing some effect. A number of cells in the brain have receptors that are highly sensitive to nicotine. This unique sensitivity to nicotine causes the drug to provide a real "hit" when it reaches the brain.

Repeated exposure to nicotine through smoking results in very rapid tolerance. That means that smokers get used to it and need increasing doses to achieve the "hit." As cigarettes are smoked, the smoker gets less and less of a psychological and physical effect. As the day wears on, and more cigarettes are smoked, people often smoke more out of habit or to avoid discomfort than for pleasure. There seems to be an internal sensing system, like a thermostat, that knows when nicotine levels are too low. Most smokers require a minimum of about ten cigarettes a day to maintain a so-called comfort zone. If too many cigarettes are smoked, the person may experience nausea and other symptoms of nicotine poisoning.

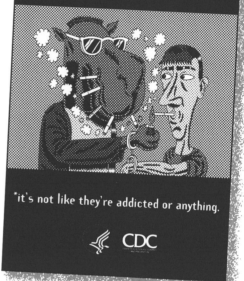

More than 80 percent of young people who smoke one pack or more of cigarettes per day report that they "need" or are dependent on cigarettes.

The younger people are when they start smoking cigarettes, the more likely they are to become strongly addicted to nicotine.

Young people who try to quit suffer the same nicotine withdrawal symptoms as adults who try to quit.

About two thirds of teenage smokers say they want to quit smoking, and more than two thirds say they would not have started smoking if they could choose again.

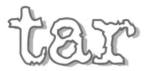

tar

Tar is not present in unburned tobacco. It is the product of organic matter burned in the presence of air and water at a sufficiently high temperature.

Tobacco products such as snuff and chew do not deliver tar, but they still contain nicotine.

Tar is one of the major hazards in cigarette smoking. It causes a variety of cancers in laboratory animals. Minute separate particles fill the tiny air-holes in the lungs and contribute to respiratory problems such as emphysema.

Cigarette manufacturers have reduced the tar in their cigarettes in an effort to provide "safer" cigarettes. Tar is important to the taste of cigarettes, however. When people smoke low-tar cigarettes, they have to inhale deeply to get the most enjoyment. That defeats the purpose of a low-tar cigarette. Ironically, cigarettes engineered to deliver low-tar results when smoked by machines deliver higher yields when smoked by people.

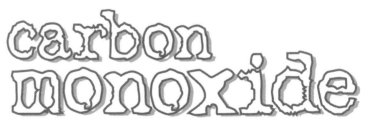

carbon monoxide

Carbon monoxide is a gas that results when materials are burned. Carbon monoxide production increases when the oxygen supply is cut back, as is the case inside a burning cigarette. Carbon monoxide is also produced by automobile engines and even by gas stoves and ovens. Smoking is like putting your mouth around the exhaust pipe of your car and breathing in.

Carbon monoxide easily passes from the tiny airholes in the lungs into the bloodstream. There carbon monoxide combines with hemoglobin. Hemoglobin is the part of the blood that normally carries carbon dioxide out of the body and oxygen back into the body. When the hemoglobin is all bound up by carbon monoxide, a shortage of oxygen may result. High levels of carbon monoxide can starve the body of oxygen. When the heart detects insufficient levels of oxygen, it may flutter. In extreme cases, heart attacks may result.

Each cigarette causes a brief boost in the body's carbon monoxide level, which lasts for a few minutes. Then the level declines until the next cigarette is smoked. However, each cigarette adds slightly to the person's overall carbon monoxide level.

Chemicals in Mainstream Tobacco Smoke

The portion of smoke pulled into the smoker's lungs from the butt end of a burning cigarette is known as mainstream smoke. Cigarette smoke is made up of both gas and solids. The unburned cigarette is comprised of many organic materials: tobacco leaves, paper products, sugars, and nicotine. It contains inorganic materials, too: water, radioactive elements, and metals. When tobacco burns, more

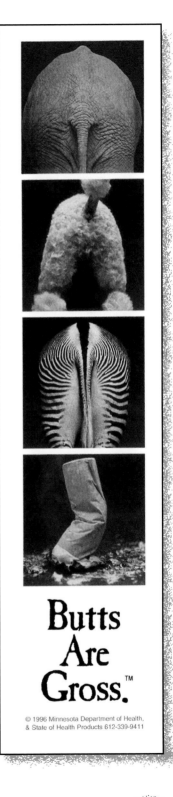

Butts Are Gross.™

© 1996 Minnesota Department of Health,
& State of Health Products 612-339-9411

Here are some of the **chemicals** smokers take in from **mainstream smoke.** A carcinogen **causes cancer.**

Carbon monoxide [auto exhaust poison]

Carbon dioxide

Carbonyl sulfide

Benzene*

Toluene [industrial solvent; in explosives]

Formaldehyde** [embalming fluid]

Acrolein [aquatic herbicide]

Acetone [poisonous solvent]

Pyridine [poisonous solvent]

3-Methylpyridine [insecticide solvent]

3-Vinylpyridine

Hydrogen cyanide [rat/insect poison]

Hydrazine [rocket fuel chemical]

Ammonia [poisonous gas, cleaning agent]

Methylamine [tanning agent]

Dimethylamine [tanning accelerator]

Nitrogen oxides

N-Nitrosodimethylamine**

N-Nitrosodiethylamine**

N-Nitrosopyrrolidine**

Formic acid [caustic solvent]

Acetic acid [caustic solvent]

Methyl chloride [poisonous refrigerant]

1,3-Butadiene**

Particulate matter [some***]

Nicotine [insecticide]

Anatabine

Phenol [toilet disinfectant]

Catechol [tanning, dyeing agent]

Hydroquinone [photographic developing agent]

Aniline** [industrial solvent]

2-Toluidine [agent in dye manufacture]

2-Napthylamine*

4-Aminobiphenyl*

Ben[a]anthracene***

Benzo[a]pyrene**

Cholesterol

y-Butyrolactone***

Quinoline [specimen preservative]

Harman

N-Nitrosonornicotine***

Cadmium**

Nickel*

Zinc [anticorrosion coating for metals]

Polonium-210* [radioactive element]

Benzoic acid [tobacco curing agent]

Lactic acid [caustic solvent]

Glycolic acid [metal cleaning agent]

Succinic acid [agent in lacquer manufacture]

PCDDs and PCDFs (dioxins, dubenzofurns)

* Known Human Carcinogen

** Probable Human Carcinogen

*** Animal Carcinogen

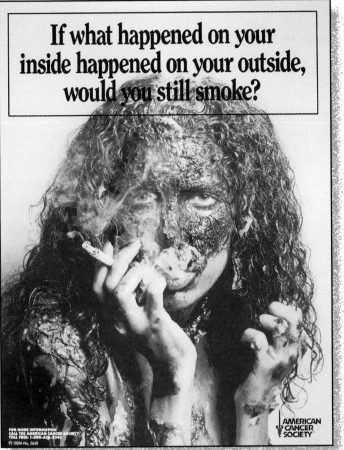

If what happened on your inside happened on your outside, would you still smoke?

FOR MORE INFORMATION
CALL THE AMERICAN CANCER SOCIETY
TOLL FREE: 1-800-ACS-2345
91-100M-No. 5648

AMERICAN
CANCER
SOCIETY

than 4,000 known compounds are created or transferred into the ash or smoke.

Sidestream Tobacco Smoke

The portion of smoke that comes off the burning end of a cigarette, pipe, or cigar between puffs is called sidestream smoke, or secondhand smoke. When a person breathes in sidestream smoke, it is called passive or involuntary smoking. The components of sidestream smoke are somewhat different from those of the mainstream smoke that smokers exhale. Sidestream smoke contains higher concentrations of certain toxic substances, including several cancer-causing ones, than mainstream smoke does.

In the United States, 50 million smokers annually smoke approximately 600 billion cigarettes, 4 billion cigars, and the equivalent of 11 billion pipes of tobacco. Since people spend approximately 90 percent of their time indoors, this means that about 467,000 tons of tobacco are burned indoors each year. Over a 16-hour day, the average smoker smokes about two cigarettes per hour, and takes about ten minutes per cigarette. Thus, it takes only a few smokers in a given space to release a more-or-less steady sidestream of smoke into the indoor air.

Many respected groups have concluded that secondhand smoke causes lung cancer. The groups include the U.S. Surgeon General's office, the National Cancer Institute, the National Research Council, the National Institute of Occupational Safety and Health, the International Agency for Research on Cancer, and the U.S. Occupational Safety and Health Administration. In 1993, the U.S. Environmental Protection Agency declared secondhand smoke a known—not just "probable" or "possible"—human carcinogen, or cancer-causing agent.

Respiratory Health Effects of Environmental Tobacco Smoke

Environmental Tobacco Smoke (ETS) is a combination of sidestream smoke given off by the smoldering cigarettes and mainstream smoke exhaled by smokers. ETS contaminates the air and is absorbed

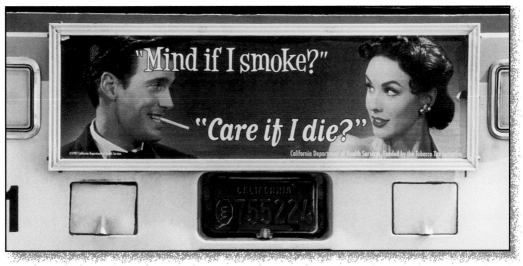

Bus poster from California

into clothing, curtains, and furniture. Although ETS is dangerous to everyone, fetuses, infants, and children are most at risk. This is because ETS can damage developing organs such as the lungs and brain.

In adults, ETS is a human lung carcinogen, responsible for approximately 3,000 lung cancer deaths in nonsmokers and 12,000 deaths from other cancers every year in the United States.

In adults, ETS has subtle but significant effects on the respiratory health of nonsmokers, including reduced lung function, increased coughing, phlegm production, and chest discomfort.

In children of all ages, ETS exposure decreases lung efficiency and impairs lung function. It increases both the frequency and severity of childhood asthma. It is estimated that 200,000 to 1,000,000 asthmatic children have their condition worsened by exposure to ETS.

In children, ETS exposure increases the likelihood of bronchitis and pneumonia. A 1992 study by the Environmental Protection Agency says that ETS is responsible for 150,000 to 300,000 lower respiratory-tract infections annually in infants and young children up to 18 months of age. These infections result in 15,000 hospitalizations.

In children, ETS exposure increases the number of ear infections they will experience. Ear infections are the most common cause of hearing loss in children.

Secondhand smoke can aggravate sinusitis, rhinitis, cystic fibrosis, coughing, and postnasal drip. It also increases the number of colds and sore throats in children.

In children who do not have asthmatic symptoms, ETS exposure puts them at risk for asthma.

Pregnant women who smoke affect the health of their babies.

Smokeless Tobacco

There are two main types of smokeless tobacco: chewing tobacco and snuff. Most smokeless tobacco is grown in Kentucky, Pennsylvania, Tennessee, Virginia, West Virginia, and Wisconsin.

Chewing tobacco comes in several forms: loose-leaf, plug, and twist.

Snuff is sold in cans and comes in three forms: moist, dry, and fine-cut. Smokeless tobacco is generally referred to as "dip," "pinch," or "chew." Users are called "chewers" or "dippers."

Moist snuff is by far the most popular form of smokeless tobacco, especially among younger chewers. It consists of articles or strips of tobacco (or packets resembling tea bags) that may be treated with flavors such as mint, menthol, and wintergreen.

People who chew tobacco place a wad of loose-leaf tobacco or a plug of compressed tobacco in the cheek. Snuff users place a small amount of powdered or finely cut tobacco (loose or wrapped in a pouch) between the gum and cheek. The user sucks on the moist mass of tobacco, called a "quid." Most dippers hold the quid in the same location in the mouth, the site where 93 percent of the primary lesions are found that lead to cancer.

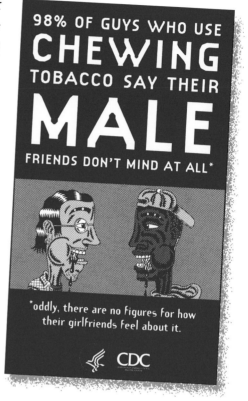

98% OF GUYS WHO USE **CHEWING** TOBACCO SAY THEIR **MALE** FRIENDS DON'T MIND AT ALL*

*oddly, there are no figures for how their girlfriends feel about it.

CDC

Loose-leaf chewing tobacco consists primarily of air-cured tobacco and, in most cases, is heavily treated with licorice and sugars. Plug tobacco is the oldest form of chewing tobacco. Plug tobacco is produced from the heavier grades of leaves harvested from the top of the plant, freed from stems, immersed in a mixture of licorice and sugar, pressed into a plug, covered by a wrapper leaf, and reshaped. Twist tobacco is made from cured burley and air- and fire-cured leaves, which are flavored and twisted to resemble a decorative rope or pigtail. Dry snuff is processed into a powdered substance that may contain flavor and aroma additives, including spices.

Chew and its juices must be disposed of periodically through spitting. The reason for spitting rather than swallowing is that tobacco juice is not considered tasty, even by tobacco addicts. In fact, it has been compared to battery acid and worse.

Smokeless tobacco is not a safe alternative to cigarettes. It causes oral cancer (cancer of the lip, tongue, cheek, jaw, or throat), gingivitis, gum recession, bad breath, and permanently stains teeth.

Oral cancer kills 50 percent of its victims within five years of diagnosis.

Here are a few of the ingredients found in spit tobacco.

Polonium 210 [nuclear waste]
N-Nitrosamines [cancer-causing compounds]
Formaldehyde [embalming fluid]
Nicotine [addictive drug]
Cadmium [used in car batteries]
Cyanide, Arsenic, Benzene, Lead [nerve poison]

Tobacco Taxation

Tobacco is taxed in a variety of ways by federal, state, and local governments.

FEDERAL TAXES: During the late 1700s and mid-1800s, the federal government experimented with taxes on tobacco products. However, because producers and consumers opposed them, the taxes were repealed. During the first half of the 1900s, federal taxes were increased to help finance U.S.

wars. In 1951, during the Korean War (1950–1953), the tax was increased from 7 to 8 cents per pack and remained at that level for the next 30 years. In 1986, the federal tax on cigarettes doubled to 16 cents per pack. But the reason was different. The taxes were raised to deal with the increasing federal budget deficit. On January 1, 1991, federal taxes on cigarettes were increased to 20 cents per pack. In 1993, federal taxes were increased to 24 cents, and in 1997 by another 10 cents per pack. Taxes are scheduled to rise 5 cents more in 2002.

STATE TAXES: In 1921, Iowa became the first state to impose an excise tax on cigarettes. In 1969, North Carolina became the last state to enact an excise tax on cigarettes. As with the federal cigarette taxes, state cigarette taxes have partly represented attempts to raise revenue rather than to lower smoking prevalence. But recently, California and Massachusetts have used large increases in cigarette taxes to fund antismoking campaigns and discourage people from smoking.

PROPOSED FEDERAL AND STATE TAXES: More and more Americans are dying from tobacco use, and smoking rates are increasing among American children. Some tobacco control policymakers feel the time has come for a major increase in federal and state tobacco excise taxes. They feel a major tobacco tax increase is a matter of life and death for hundreds of thousands, if not millions, of Americans. By conservative estimates, a $2-per-pack tax increase would reduce the number of people who smoke and prevent millions of premature tobacco-caused deaths over time. Raising taxes is the most effective way to reduce tobacco use among young people. Canada proved prices influence young people's consumption of tobacco. Between 1981 and 1991, Canada raised tobacco taxes by nearly $3 (U.S.) per pack, and youth smoking declined in that country by more than 60 percent. Many lawmakers in the Democratic and Republican parties favor raising tobacco taxes to help fund health care reform and to balance the federal budget.

State Cigarette Taxes
cents/pack
(as of October 1, 1997)

Alaska	100	Florida	33.9
Hawaii	100	South Dakota	33.0
California	87.0	Pennsylvania	31.0
Washington	82.5	Idaho	28.0
New Jersey	80.0	New Hampshire	25.0
Massachusetts	76.0	Delaware	24.0
Michigan	75.0	Kansas	24.0
Maine	74.0	Ohio	24.0
Rhode Island	71.0	Oklahoma	23.0
Oregon	68.0	New Mexico	21.0
Maryland	66.0	Colorado	20.0
Washington, D.C.	65.0	Louisiana	20.0
Wisconsin	59.0	Mississippi	18.0
Arizona	58.0	Montana	18.0
Illinois	58.0	Missouri	17.0
New York	56.0	West Virginia	17.0
New Hampshire	52.0	Alabama	16.5
Utah	51.5	Indiana	15.5
Connecticut	50.0	Tennessee	13.0
Minnesota	48.0	Georgia	12.0
North Dakota	44.0	Wyoming	12.0
Vermont	44.0	South Carolina	7.0
Texas	41.0	North Carolina	5.0
Iowa	36.0	Kentucky	3.0
Nevada	35.0	Virginia	2.5
Nebraska	34.0		

State Laws Legislated on Tobacco Issues (1994)

RESTRICTIONS ON SMOKING IN PUBLIC PLACES: Forty-eight states and the District of Columbia have some restrictions. These laws range from simple, limited prohibitions, such as restrictions in schools, to laws that limit or ban smoking in virtually all public places. These places include elevators, public buildings, health facilities, public conveyances, museums, shopping malls, retail stores, and educational facilities. The most extensive clean indoor air laws–Utah and California—include restaurants and private workplaces.

TOBACCO EXCISE TAXES: All 50 states and the District of Columbia impose an excise tax on cigarettes, ranging from a high of $.825 per pack in Washington to a low of $.025 per pack in Virginia.

SMOKELESS TOBACCO: Forty states have excise taxes on smokeless tobacco products, including chewing tobacco and snuff.

AGE RESTRICTIONS ON SALES OF TOBACCO PRODUCTS: All 50 states and the District of Columbia prohibit the sale of tobacco products to minors. Most states define minors as persons under 18 years of age. Three states—Alabama, Alaska, and Utah—define minors as persons under 19 years of age. Pennsylvania requires individuals to be 21 years old or older to buy cigarettes, but 18 for other tobacco purchases.

RESTRICTIONS ON DISTRIBUTION OF TOBACCO PRODUCT SAMPLES: Thirty-eight

143

states restrict the distribution of free samples of tobacco products.

RESTRICTIONS ON SALES OF TOBACCO PRODUCTS IN VENDING MACHINES: Twenty-eight states and the District of Columbia restrict the sale of tobacco products in vending machines.

LICENSING REQUIREMENTS: Forty-one states and the District of Columbia require the licensing of parties that sell tobacco products.

Stadiums that Ban Tobacco Ads

Oriole Park at Camden Yards, Baltimore

Fenway Park, Boston

Wrigley Field, Chicago

Jacobs Field, Cleveland

Coors Field, Denver

Astrodome, Houston

Kauffman Stadium, Kansas City

Dodger Stadium, Los Angeles

Hubert H. Humphrey Metrodome, Minneapolis

Olympic Stadium, Montreal

Oakland-Almeda County Coliseum, Oakland, California

Veterans Stadium, Philadelphia

America West Arena, Phoenix

Three Rivers Stadium, Pittsburgh

Busch Stadium, St. Louis

Qualcomm Stadium, San Diego

Kingdome, Seattle

The Ballpark, Arlington, Texas

SkyDome, Toronto

The Delta Center, Salt Lake City

Dasherboards of all NHL rinks

All Olympic stadiums

Selected Sports Stadiums That Are Smoke-Free

The Ballpark—Texas

Brown County Veterans Memorial Stadium—Wisconsin

Jacobs Field, Ohio

Continental Airlines Arena—New Jersey
   (during family shows)

Giants Stadium—New Jersey

Mile High Stadium—Colorado

Madison Square Garden—New York

Spartan Stadium—Michigan State University,
   East Lansing, Michigan

The Target Center—Minneapolis, Minnesota

Oakland-Almeda County Coliseum—California

Ohio Stadium, Ohio State University—Columbus, Ohio

Beaver Stadium Pennsylvania State University—
   State College, Pennsylvania

Providence Civic Center, Rhode Island

Kingdome, Seattle, Washington

Stanford Stadium, Stanford University, California

USAir Arena—Landover, Maryland
   smoking is restricted to one area of concourse

The Delta Center, Salt Lake City, Utah

Mountaineer Field, West Virginia University—
   Morgantown, West Virginia
   restricted to designated areas

*Every Major League Baseball stadium has smoke-free
seating areas

APPENDIX TWO

RESOURCES

Top-Ten Tobacco Videos for Youth

There are dozens and dozens of videos about tobacco. Stop Teenage Addiction to Tobacco (STAT) came up with this list based on its experience showing videos to youngsters. Here's STAT's top-ten list of videos.

1. **"SAY GOOD-BYE, CAMEL JOE"**
   Running time—8 minutes.
   For Grades 5 and up.
   Distributed by STAT, Springfield, MA.
   1-413-732-7828.

2. **"TAKE ACTION! Teen Voices for Change"**
   Running time—20 minutes. For Grades 9–12.
   Produced by the Stanford Center for Research in Disease Prevention. Available through STAT.

3. **"STOP THE SALE, PREVENT THE ADDICTION"**
   Running time—26 minutes. For Grades 7 and up. Distributed by the Office on Smoking and Health, National Center for Chronic Disease Prevention and Health Promotion, Centers for Disease Control, Atlanta, Georgia. 1-800-CDC-1311.

4. **"THE TRUTH ABOUT TOBACCO"**
   Running time—17 minutes. For Grades 7–12.
   Distributed by Syndistar, Inc.
   St. Rose, Louisiana.
   1-504-468-1100.

5. **"AD-LIBBING IT"**
   Running time—18 minutes. For Grades 6 and up.
   Distributed by Comprehensive Health
   Education Foundation, Seattle, Washington.
   1-208-824-2907.

6. **"TOBACCO FREE, YOU & ME"***
   Running time—19 minutes. For Grades 5 and up.

7. **"SMOKE SCREEN"***
   Running time—20 minutes. For Grades 7–12.

8. **"SMOKELESS TOBACCO: Spittin' Image"***
   Running time—14 minutes. For Grades 7–12.
   Washington, D.C.
   1-800-536-6843.

9. **"WHAT'S WRONG WITH TOBACCO"**
   Running time—30 minutes.
   For Grades 8–12. Distributed by
   Human Relations Media, Inc.
   1-800-431-2050.

10. **"CALIFORNIA DREAMS:
    Harley and the Marlboro Man"**
    Running time—30 minutes.
    For Grades 8-12.
    Produced for NBC
    by Peter Engell Productions, Inc.
    Distributed by the Office on Smoking and Health,
    National Center for Chronic Disease Prevention
    and Health Promotion, Centers for Disease Control,
    Atlanta, Georgia. 1-800-CDC-1311.

*Distributed by Durrin Productions, Inc.

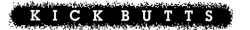
Tobacco Control: Government Agencies

Centers for Disease Control and Prevention
Office on Smoking and Health
Distributes smoking and health information in a variety of forms including pamphlets, posters, scientific reports, and public-service announcements. Keeps track of smoking-related deaths each year and epidemiological information on who smokes, broken down by age, income, and race. Produces the annual Surgeon General's report on tobacco. Puts out a bulletin, *Morbidity and Mortality Weekly Report (MMWR),* which sometimes contains tobacco studies.

Centers for Disease Control and Prevention
National Center for Chronic Disease Prevention and Health Promotion, Office on Smoking and Health
Mailstop K-50
4770 Buford Highway, NE
Atlanta, GA 30341-3724/(770) 488–5705
(General information and publication requests)
Internet: **http://www.cdc.gov/tobacco**

Bureau of Alcohol, Tobacco, and Firearms
Provides general information about current tax rates and tax revenues regarding tobacco.
U.S. Department of the Treasury
Bureau of Alcohol, Tobacco, and Firearms
Distilled Spirits and Tobacco Branch
650 Massachusetts Avenue, NW
Washington, DC 20226/(202) 927–8210
Internet: **http://www.atf.treas.gov/**

Environmental Protection Agency (EPA)
Provides publications and information on the harmful effects of environmental tobacco smoke and indoor air pollution. Provides consumer information on ways to minimize exposure to tobacco smoke.
Environmental Protection Agency
Indoor Air Quality Information Clearinghouse
P.O. Box 37133
Washington, DC 20013–7133
(202) 233–9315—Indoor Air Division
Internet: **http://www.epa.gov/**

Federal Trade Commission (FTC)
Provides publications and information related to tobacco advertising and trade policies. Oversees warning labels, advertising, and advertising expenditures. Keeps track of nicotine and tar in cigarettes.
Federal Trade Commission
601 Pennsylvania Avenue, NW
Washington, DC 20580
(202) 326–2222—publications
(202) 326–3150—tobacco-related questions
Internet: **http://www.ftc.gov/index.html**

Food and Drug Administration (FDA)
Wants to regulate nicotine in tobacco as a drug . It already regulates other products containing nicotine such as patches, gum, and other aids to quitting smoking.
Food and Drug Administration
5600 Fishers Lane HF1
Rockville, MD 20857/(301) 443–1130
Toll-free: 1-888-FDA-4KIDS (for publications)
Internet: **http://www.fda.gov**

National Cancer Institute
Provides publications and provides information for the public about cancer or quitting from its Cancer Information Service. Has leaflets about spit tobacco.
National Cancer Institute
Building 31, Room 10A24
9000 Rockville Pike
Bethesda, MD 20892
Toll-free: 1-800-4-CANCER
Internet: **http://www.nci.nih.gov/**

National Clearinghouse for Alcohol and Drug Information
Provides information about the health risks of using addictive drugs including tobacco. Information is available in various forms including videos, fact sheets, posters, and pamphlets.
Center for Substance Abuse Prevention
National Clearinghouse for
Alcohol and Drug Information
P.O. Box 2345
Rockville, MD 20847-2345/(301) 468–2600
Toll-free: 1–800–Say–No–To
Internet: **http://www.health.org/youth.htm**

U.S. Department of Agriculture
Provides information related to agricultural issues pertaining to tobacco. Keeps track of domestic production, policy, trade, economics, and consumption. Publishes a statistical report: "Tobacco: Situation and Outlook."
United States Department of Agriculture
Tobacco and Peanut Division
Room 5750 South Building
P.O. Box 2415
Washington, DC 20013/(202)720-2791
Internet: **http://www.usda.gov/**

State and local health departments
Provide a variety of smoking and health information to the public. Check the government section of your phone book for current addresses and phone numbers.

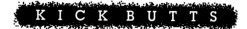

NonProfit Organizations

Action on Smoking and Health

Produces materials on a variety of smoking and health topics for the public, with emphasis on legal action to protect nonsmokers' health. It pursues suits on smoking control issues such as minors' access to vending machines, secondhand smoke, smoke-free workplaces, restaurants, transportation, and custody issues. (Its director, John Banzhaf III, played a key role in getting legislation passed to make national airline flights smoke-free and to get tobacco ads off the airwaves.) Newsletter.

Action on Smoking and Health
2013 H Street, NW
Washington, DC 20006/(202) 659–4310; http://ash.org

The Advocacy Institute

Works on efforts to counter the influence of the tobacco industry and consults on policy issues related to tobacco control. The Institute manages SCARCNET, a computer network for tobacco control advocates.

The Advocacy Institute
1730 Rhode Island Avenue, NW, Suite 600
Washington, DC 20036–4505/(202) 659–8475; http://www.advocacy.org

American Academy of Otolaryngology

Provides leaflets about spit tobacco and secondhand smoke.

American Academy of Otolaryngology
Head and Neck Surgery Foundation
One Prince Street/Alexandria, VA 22314

American Cancer Society (ACS)

Provides smoking education, prevention, and quitting programs and distributes pamphlets, posters, and other materials on smoking. It sponsors the Great American Smokeout, an annual event in November. Look in your phone book for a local ACS office in your area.

American Cancer Society (National Headquarters)
1599 Clifton Road, NE
Atlanta, GA 30329/1–800–ACS–2345; http//www.cancer.org

American Council on Science and Health (ACSH)

Provides scientific evaluations on tobacco-related topics. Its journal, *Priorities*, has readable articles on tobacco issues. During the 1980s, ACSH did a number of surveys of magazines and tobacco advertising. Its director, Elizabeth Whelan, has been writing about the tobacco industry for years.

American Council on Science and Health
1995 Broadway, 2nd floor
New York, NY 10023–5860/(212) 362–7044

American Heart Association (AHA)

Promotes smoking intervention programs at schools, workplaces, and health care sites. Look in your phone book for a local AHA chapter in your area.

American Heart Association National Center
7272 Greenville Avenue
Dallas, TX 65231
(214) 373–7300/1–800–242–8721; http://www.amhrt.org

American Lung Association (ALA)

Conducts programs addressing smoking cessation, prevention, and the protection of nonsmokers' health and provides a variety of educational materials for the public and health professionals. Look in your phone book for a local ALA chapter in your area.
American Lung Association
1740 Broadway
New York, NY 10019–4274
(212) 315–8700/1–800–586–4872; http://www.lung.usa.org

Americans for Nonsmokers Rights (ANR)

Provides information to organizations and individuals to assist in passing ordinances, implementing workplace regulations, and developing smoking policies in the workplace. Active on local, state, and national levels. Also works on advertising and youth access. Projects includes "Teens as Teachers." Newsletter.
Americans for Nonsmokers Rights
2530 San Pablo Avenue, Suite J
Berkeley, CA 94702/(510) 841–3032; http://www.no-smoke.org

Doctors Ought to Care (DOC)

Provides school curricula, smoking prevention information, and tobacco counteradvertisements for use in clinics, classrooms, and communities. Newsletter.
Doctors Ought to Care
5510 Greenbriar, Suite 235
Houston, TX 77005/(713) 798–7729

Group Against Smokers' Pollution (GASP)

Provides educational materials and information and referral services concerning the health hazards of secondhand smoke and the establishment of nonsmoking laws and policies.
Group Against Smokers' Pollution
P.O. Box 632
College Park, MD 20740/(301) 459–4791

SmokeFree Educational Services, Inc.

Works for smoke-free air in public places through local, state, and federal legislation. Provides smoking and health educational materials for schools and workplaces in the form of booklets, posters, videos, and stickers. Sponsored children's smoke-free ad contests. Newsletter.
SmokeFree Educational Services, Inc.
375 South End Avenue, Suite 32F
New York, NY 10280/(212) 912–0960; http.//www.smokefree.org

Stop Teenage Addiction to Tobacco (STAT)

Works to regulate advertising and promotions and to heighten public awareness of industry marketing practices that may target young people. Seeks to restrict cigarette vending machines and support smoke-free community ordinances. www.stat.org

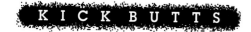

Stop Teenage Addiction to Tobacco
511 E. Columbus Avenue
Springfield, MA 01105/(413) 732–7828

Tobacco Products Liability Project
Provides information on lawsuits against tobacco companies and class-action suits alleging that tobacco companies knew more about the addictive nature of nicotine than they admit. Newsletter.
Tobacco Products Liability Project
Northeastern University School of Law
400 Huntington Avenue
Boston, MA 02155/(617) 373–2026

World Health Organization (WHO)
United Nations agency provides information through its Tobacco Free Initiative. Looks at Youth and Tobacco (with links to other youth sites) and the annual World No-Tobacco Day (May 31).
World Health Organization
2 United Nations Plaza/DC-2 Building
New York, NY 10017/(212) 223-2920; http://tobacco.who.int

Tobacco Use Prevention and Control Programs

American Legacy Foundation
A national, independent, public charity established by the November 1998 Master Settlement Agreement, ALF supports a truth campaign—a national youth movement against the tobacco industry, research on tobacco issues, grants to states, and organizations to develop grassroots youth empowerment programs, technical assistance and training on youth empowerment, counter-marketing, cessation, and policy formation.
American Legacy Foundation
1001 G Street, NW, Suite 800
Washington, DC 20001/(202) 454-5555; www.americanlegacy.org

National Center for Tobacco-Free Kids
A national organization, also known as the Campaign for Tobacco-Free Kids, is a non-governmental, inclusive organization that works to prevent tobacco use by children and youth. It provides the public with facts sheets and special reports, presents Youth Advocates of the Year awards, and sponsors Kick Butts Day.
National Center for Tobacco-Free Kids
17-7 L Street NW, Suite #800
Washington, DC 20036/(202) 296-5469; www.tobaccofreekids.org

SmokeLess States Program (American Medical Association/Robert Wood Johnson Foundation)
The SmokeLess States program, a large non-governmental program, funds 30 state-wide coalitions that promote public awareness of the dangers of tobacco use and pursue local prevention and treatment programs.
American Medical Association (National Headquarters)
515 North State Street
Chicago, Illinois 60610/(312) 464-5000; www.ama-assn.org/special/aos

BIBLIOGRAPHY

This bibliography is for smoke-free activists. It will help you find how-to books and locate organizations to write for more information to help you plan smoke-free activities.

ACTIVISM 2000 PROJECT, *Youth-Produced PSAs: TV Messages That Matter* (video and guide). P.O. Box E. Kensington, MD 20895. Kids have been taking to the airwaves and creating PSAs to highlight issues that affect their generation. The ACTIVISM 2000 PROJECT, a clearinghouse dedicated to encouraging young people to be participants in shaping public policies, has put together an eight-minute video. The video features brief but dynamic messages that demonstrate how kids can capture the attention of peers and policymakers alike. A companion book, *Pointers About Public Service Announcements,* describes how to create a hard-hitting PSA that gets on television and radio. Other materials are also available.

Americans for Nonsmokers' Rights Foundation (ANRF). *How to Butt In: Teens Take Action Guidebook.* Berkeley, CA: ANRF, 1995. This booklet provides guidance on "How to Make the Tobacco Industry Butt Out of Your Life." It shows how to write letters to city officials and newspapers, write press releases, create public-service announcements, and other things you need to know to be a social activist.

Boy Scouts of America, Drug Abuse Task Force, 1325 W. Walnut Hill Lane, P.O. Box 152079, Irving, TX 75015-2079. The Boy Scouts have a program called *Don't Be Tricked by Drugs: A Deadly Game* that includes a variety of material about tobacco. Write for information.

Boys and Girls Clubs of America, 1230 W. Peachtree Street, NW, Atlanta, GA 30309-3447. This organization has a program called "SMART Moves," to help young people resist alcohol, tobacco, and other drugs. Write for information about "Start SMART," a program for girls and boys 10 to 12, and "Stay SMART," for young people 13 to 15, plus other programs.

Girls, Incorporated, National Resource Center, 441 West Michigan Avenue, Indianapolis, IN 46202. Write for information about "Friendly PEERsuasion," a substance abuse prevention program for girls 11 to 14.

Institute of Medicine. *Growing Up Tobacco Free: Preventing Nicotine Addiction in Children and Youths*. Washington, D.C.: National Academy Press, 1994. This report deals with kids and tobacco use, but it's really aimed at adults. Each chapter offers recommendations for public action. Special features include the cover and the posters appearing throughout the book. They come from Andrew Tobias's book *Kids Say Don't Smoke*. (Also check out the Surgeon General's report about youth under "U.S. Department of Health and Human Services.")

Lesko, Wendy Schaetzel. *No Kidding Around! America's Young Activists Are Changing Our World and You Can Too*. Kensington, MD: Information USA, Inc., 1992. The title says it all. The handbook on civic activism by kids includes a few stories about kids fighting tobacco. "Never underestimate the power of your voice," said Lynn Terrill of Massachusetts, a student who helped launch a successful tobacco-free schools campaign. This book has great suggestions for mapping out smoke-free campaigns.

Lewis, Barbara A. *The Kid's Guide to Social Action*. Minneapolis, MN: Free Spirit Publishing, Inc., 1991. This book includes stories about real kids making a difference and offers guides to honing skills such as telephoning, letter writing, interviewing, speech making, surveying, petitioning, proposal writing, fund-raising, advertising, and so on. There's a section on changing laws and a terrific collection of resources and 20 ready-to-copy-and-use social action forms.

Tobias, Andrew. *Kids Say Don't Smoke*. New York: Workman Publishing, 1991. A selection of prize-winning posters by New York City kids show the dangers of smoking, plus written facts. Many of the posters in *Kids Say Don't Smoke* have appeared in other books, on T-shirts, and in subway stations.

U.S. Department of Health and Human Services (DHHS). *Preventing Tobacco Use Among Young People: A Report of the Surgeon General*. Atlanta, GA: DHHS, Public Health Service, Centers for Disease Control and Prevention, Office on Smoking and Health, 1994. This report focuses on young people 10 through 18. The report examines decades of scientific literature on the factors that influence kids to start using tobacco. It discusses the advertising and promotional activities of the tobacco industry. It reviews research on the effects of these activities on young people. The report also deals with the health consequences of tobacco use by young people.

WRS Group, Inc. *Health Edco* (Catalog). In the tobacco section of this catalog are lists of books, videos, posters, folding displays, charts, overhead transparencies, balloons, and buttons with antismoking messages. There are models of healthy and unhealthy lungs. There are mechanical smokes that show the collection of tar in lungs or the dangers of secondhand smoke. This company sells "Mr. Gross Mouth™" and "Mr. Dip Lip™." Both show the effects of using smokeless tobacco.

ACKNOWLEDGMENTS

I hope each of you who sees his or her name on this list hears me applauding you. This book could not have been done without the materials you sent, the phone calls you returned, and the faxes you promptly transmitted. My thanks to you all for enriching this book with your priceless expertise.

John Banzhaf III, Executive Director of Action on Smoking and Health, Washington, D.C.; Lynn Carol Birgmann, Coordinator, Kentucky Youth for Healthy Futures, Louisville, Kentucky; Tricia Brazil, American Nonsmokers' Rights Foundation, Berkeley, California; Joe Cherner, President, SmokeFree Educational Services, Inc., New York, New York; Kim Contardi, Tobacco Control Resource Center, San Diego County, California; Annette W. Curtis, Reference Librarian, Mid-Continent Public Library, Genealogy and Local History, Independence, Missouri; Ronald J. Des Roches, Crimson Properties, Inc., Ashland, Virginia; Susie "D" Dickman, "Chicago 4" friend and my eyes and ears in the Midwest; Alfred Epstein, Librarian, Frances E. Willard Memorial Library, Evanston, Illinois; Jim Ferguson, Little League, Williamsport, Pennsylvania; Susie "G" Gottlieb, "Chicago 4" friend and researcher extraordinaire; Suzanne Greenwald, Highland Park, Illinois; Nancy Halbig, Assistant to Richard L. Bender, Roundup, Montana; Adam Hirschfelder; Joann Hoffman, M.P.H., El Progreso del Disierto, Inc., Coachella, California; Ann Marie Holen, Alaska Native Health Board, Anchorage, Alaska; Alyonik Hrushow, M.P.H., Tobacco Control Project Director, County of San Francisco, California; Dr. John S. Katsoulis, Assistant Superintendent, Instruction, Billerica Public Schools, Billerica, Massachusetts; Ronald Klempner; Wendy Schaetzel Lesko, Executive Director, Activism 2000 Project, Kensington, Maryland; Mary Levey, Girl Scouts of the U.S.A., New York, New York; Aunt Shirley Litt; Anita E. Manning, Healthy Schools Coordinator, Harrison County Schools, Clarksburg, West Virginia; Annette Marley, Alaska Native Health Board, Trampling Tobacco Project; Anchorage Alaska; Laurie Michel; Susan K. Morgan, Coordinator, Marion County Tobacco Control Coalition, Fairmont, West Virginia; Brigid Olson, Escondido Community Health Center, Escondido, California; Denise Otkins, Stop Teenage Addiction to Tobacco (STAT), Springfield, Massachusetts; Mickey Pearlman; Thi Pham, State Tobacco Program Coordinator, Asian Health Services, Oakland, California; Marvin Rayfield, Lucy Richardson, Nurse, Pine Forest Elementary School, Humble, Texas; Barbara Rochon, Operations Manager, Stop Teenage Addiction to Tobacco (STAT), Springfield, Massachusetts; Joni Rooth, "Chicago 4" friend and my eyes and ears in Texas; Pam Rutt, Vice President, Public Relations, Marvel Entertainment Group, Inc., New York, New York; Pam Schreiber, WRS Group, Inc., Waco, Texas; John Serpentelli, Animator, Philadelphia, Pennsylvania; Wynn Ava Sherron, Teacher, Heath High School, West Paducah, Kentucky; Don Shopland, Coordinator, Smoking and Tobacco Control Program, National Cancer Institute, Bethesda, Maryland; Jill Sinclair, Statewide Coordinator, ASSIST, Indiana; John Slade, M.D., Department of Medicine, St. Peter's Medical Center, New Brunswick, New Jersey; Jill O. Stewart, Nobacco News Editor, SmokeLess States Program, American Medical Association, Chicago, Illinois; Frances R. Toone, American Lung Association, New York, New York; Nereida Torres, American Lung Association, New York, New York; Marge White, Coalition for a Smoke-Free Virginia, Richmond, Virginia

The Author

INDEX

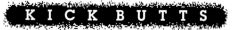

ABOUT THE AUTHOR

Arlene Hirschfelder is the author of four recent publications in the field of tobacco and has done consulting work and created curriculum in the tobacco field for both Scholastic, Inc. and Columbia University School of Social Work. Besides her passion for historical research and libraries, she enjoys drawing and gardening. Arlene is the mother of Brooke and Adam and lives in northern New Jersey.

CREDITS